"Bookstores are filled with thousands of '
hold The Secret to a leaner, stronger, hea.
The reason there are so many titles i
none of these books has the answer.

Unleash Your Alpha is different. It is the first book I've seen that addresses all aspects of a strong, healthy, productive man – nutrition, exercise, style, sex appeal, confidence, brotherhood – every part of the Great Man we all want to be (and what women want us to be).

If you're a man in search of guidance from the inside out, or if you're a woman looking for something to really improve the health and well being of your mate, you can do no better than Unleash Your Alpha."

BRYAN KRAHN,
EDITOR AND COACH, BRYANKRAHN.COM

"Most books on the subject of being a better man are centred around getting laid more and most workout books are filled with superficial solutions and sold on fear and emotion. They're directed towards the pick-up artist community and meant to be sold to 20 year old boys who aren't yet men. This book is catered towards men who want to become gentlemen.

In Mike's words, "we men have bigger waistlines than ever, soaring rates of disease, and worrying statistics for divorce, job satisfaction, depression, and suicide" – Unleash Your Alpha is a major step to reverse this trend."

JON GOODMAN,
2 X AUTHOR & CREATOR OF THE PERSONAL TRAINER DEVELOPMENT CENTRE

"Mike is a true Alpha who unequivocally walks his talk. Unleash Your Alpha is full of sage advice across a whole range of areas, each of which Mike has himself traversed, experimented, learned and applied. If you're a man and want to be the man you were born to be, get a copy of Mike's book. If you're a woman and want the man in your life to reach his potential, buy him a copy. You'll both be happy you did!"

JOHN BROADBENT,
AUTHOR MAN UNPLUGGED- EXPLORING CONTEMPORARY MASCULINITY

"Redefine what being an "alpha male" really means. Fun read! A good start to revamp your lifestyle."

DR SPENCER NADOLSKY MD,
PRACTITIONER & DIRECTOR EXAMINE.COM

"I was worried that this would just be another run of the books on health and fitness. Not to be... This is an upfront no-holds barred clear instruction manual on how to be the best man you can be. This isn't a "fluffy" read. It's direct, in your face and tells it how it is. I also appreciated that it wasn't just about the physical aspects of being an Alpha. I particularly appreciated the sections on mental and emotional well-being. If you want to know how to become the best man you can be – check this out. You won't be disappointed."

DAVE LIOW,
LECTURER, EXERCISE PHYSIOLOGIST & COACH

"Working hard building a business I took my eye off the ball of the other essentials of being a man. My fitness dropped, and so did my health, then so did my energy, then so did everything else. Mike's book pulled no punches and pointed out the truth; I had the constitution of a pink flamingo. I turned the pages and there were the answers. Unlike other books I'd read on 'fitness' or 'health' Mike took things to a new level. With a complete absence of machismo that you may expect if you misinterpret the title, this book combines humour with insights so accurate I couldn't hide from reality. More importantly, Mike simplifies the solution into an easily actionable method that that I could fit into my life (which is, and will remain relatively dominated by work). I feel better, I look better, I eat better and I have tapped into a grounded power and confidence that I'm bringing to every aspect of my life. No excuses boys.
    Man up. Read this book. The world is waiting."

GLEN CARLSON,
DIRECTOR KEY PERSON OF INFLUENCE

"Unleash Your Alpha *literally breaks down all aspects of focus and direction, building muscle, losing fat and how to build attraction into step by step frameworks that couldn't be easier to take action on. If becoming the love child of Arnold Schwarzenegger, Ghandi and Neil Strauss is something you aspire to become this book is for you."

CHRIS WREN,
THEFITNESSARCHETYPE.COM

"*Slow clap* ... Mike, this is truly amazing – kind of blown away by the quality of it. Your effort over the last 18 months has obviously paid off big time."

JAMES GARLAND,
FITANDSTRONGDADS.COM

UNLEASH YOUR
ALPHA

MIKE CAMPBELL

*To my amazing parents who laid the stones
for the path I now walk.*

Mum, you'll always be missed, but continue to inspire me.

———

*And to Nards, without you this simply wouldn't even be an idea.
You have made me into the man – the Alpha – that I am today,
continually challenging me to grow.*

My queen, my rock, my fire.

CONTENTS

FOREWORD

Mike Campbell eats, sleeps, breathes and truly lives his philosophy. He is without a doubt a proud, walking, talking, living Alpha male. The content of this inspiring book is a reflection of his truly wise ideology and it is indeed the ultimate hand book to provide you with the tools to discover your own unsurpassed physical, mental and spiritual ALPHA potential!

When I read the pages that follow I couldn't help but feel like Mike was a modern day William Wallace (from the movie *Braveheart*), urging men to join him and bellowing, "Are you with me in this battle against mediocrity?!". And at the end of the day, that's what this book opens your eyes to, the fact that life is to be lived and why not do the best darn job you can and have the best darn time while you're doing it.

Unleash Your Alpha couldn't be more punctual because let's face it, the time has definitely arrived to discard the weak, gimmicky, diet, self help and exercise books of old and return to our roots as authentic, primal ALPHA MALES! It's true, there's no denying that men over the years have unfortunately lost touch with their innate selves and taken on misguided stereotypical alpha male attributes such as arrogant, closed minded, controlling, macho and aggressive behaviours (you know the ones I'm talking about), but in truth none of those traits have any connection with the true essence that is Alpha. What Mike has managed to cleverly articulate in this book is a well rounded, informative template containing the nourishing components to guide us back to our empowered, ancestral roots!

Now, I'm a chef and I love a good recipe, so to me it's paramount that Mike's enthusiastic curiosity on how to live an extraordinary life on all levels, has led him to seek out the best ingredients to make a man.

He has studied and learned from experts across the board like exercise physiologists, anthropologists, physicians, psychiatrists, nutritionists, food scientists, fellow trainers and evolutionary biologists in order to write his well researched formula for genuine alpha living, so rest assured his advice is bang on!!!

By the time you finish this book you will have a much clearer understanding of the big picture, so get excited, grab your destiny with your own two hands and turn the page to UNLEASH YOUR ALPHA!

Pete Evans
Chef, author, father, surfer and Alpha...
Cook with Love & Laughter!

INTRODUCTION

WHAT'S THIS ALL ABOUT?

"Men are born to succeed, not to fail"

– HENRY DAVID THOREAU

Modern society has seen a shift in what it means to be male, and it's not for the better.

Look around any public space and assess the males you see. Notice any real men? The men we all want to be – strong, confident, healthy, and masculine?

Sadly, what you'll see is scores of de-conditioned and overweight men that lack energy and confidence. As a result, the rest of their life suffers – home, work, and their social lives.

Deep down we know we can be better, but pride and ego often prevent us from doing anything about it. Progress is stunted all the more by an overwhelming amount of conflicting and confusing information about how and what it takes to be a man.

Man, provider, leader – there are many terms to define the masculine half of our species, but one of the most popular is the very misconstrued idiom, *Alpha Male*.

Alpha Male used to simply mean "one who led" – it has become synonymous with arrogant, macho "blokey blokes."

So instead of a man with compassion and integrity, one who knows who he is and carries himself accordingly, we see an inwardly insecure man who feels the need for one-upmanship and dick-swinging bravado.

It's easy to see the difference between these two contrasting pictures of man.

We'll delve deeper into the new and true description of the modern Alpha, the Alpha I'm determined to see flourish, but for now I challenge you to ponder this: what man do you want to be?

Or, if you're reading this for the man in your life, what man sounds like the one to spend time with, to work for, to provide for your family, to role model for your children? The macho dickhead? The overweight and spineless mouse with low self esteem?

If either of these aren't who you want to be, then this book is for you.

In other words, if you want to be the original "Alpha male" – radiating true masculine energy, in-shape, full of subtle confidence, happy and healthy and comfortable in his skin, then this book is for you, or the men in your life.

So who am I to make these judgments about the male species? My name is Michael Campbell, and I'm a man, have been all my life. Well, once I grew out of the awkward slightly gangly and fluctuating voice teenage phase.

Not only am I a man, I'm a personal trainer and nutrition coach. I've worked closely with hundreds of men in the health and fitness industry for close to a decade.

I'm also a complete training and nutrition geek. I love researching, reading, and finding solutions to everyday problems that my clients face. I like to think of myself as a logical, perceptive guy who has gathered insight and great understanding of the troubles us modern men face.

My experience, research, and observations have led me to an inescapable conclusion: *we men can no longer work out how to be men.*

What changes do we need to make to reclaim our male identity? Who to role model? What foods to eat? How to exercise? How to make positive changes in our attitude? What to say so we don't put our foot in it? Even how to manage our time so we're not constantly so busy? We're confused about how to live life!

Do any of these issues ring true?

There's a drastic decline in the number of men even remotely resembling the original Alpha. Where are the role models for our developing male population? Where are the strong and desirable lovers, partners, and providers?

Look around – can you see the expanding waistlines and the declining health of the male population? This may very well be *you*. There's many aspects to being a man and in today's frantically paced world, with others constantly stepping into our space and pushing their wishes upon us, it's hard to get any clarity as to what kind of man you are.

I don't say this to offend or point the finger – this is more an assessment of men worldwide. For some this will come as a shock because there's little or no mainstream recognition that a problem even exists.

That's why I hold the mirror up through these pages and why I bring not only the simple solutions, but also the problem to light. We need to know, we need to admit it, and we need to address it, or we face a rapid decline into a world of weak, unhappy, fat, slow, and uninspiring men.

***

During my years of experience as a physical trainer, nutrition coach and man, I've seen the same problems forming repeatedly when it comes to men wanting to be a better version of themselves.

But all's not lost. I've developed a structure that's helped many men to change their lives and completely turn their worlds around. That's exactly what this book is about.

This system uses the latest research, proven best practices, and endless self-experimentation (plus experimentation on actual humans, *my clients*) and simplified them, establishing an easy to follow blueprint for success.

Whether it's:
- Losing fat and the "spare tyre".
- Consistently having great energy, confidence, and virility.
- Simply being able to *and wanting to*, have regular
  sex and sleep better at night.

This simple step by step plan will guide your way to balancing your hormones, getting in banging shape, and turning you into a *true* Alpha male – a man with heart *and* backbone. This will help you unleash your own *Alpha* and nail down your A-game as *the best man you can be*.

So what prevents us from finding our A-game, getting lean and muscular, and leading a life full of awesome moments? From my experience and research there are many common problems, however, the following often lead to failure or no attempt at all. These include:

- A lack of direction and desire to commit to a better lifestyle.
- Confusion over what we should eat, including when
  and how much.
- Confusion over how often we should train and what
  exactly we should do.

- Lack of knowledge and awareness around other key lifestyle factors such as sleep and stress and how crucial they are to our end goals.
- Lack of work-life balance.
- Pride and ego preventing admission of a problem to begin with and subsequent suffering in silence while problems exacerbate.
- Finally, and perhaps most importantly, a hormonal profile that a female pink flamingo would be ashamed of! This is usually a combination of all the above and at the same time a *cause* of the above. A vicious cycle of low sex drive, moobs (man boobs), body fat, and shitty self worth.

Any of these sound familiar?

So how do we overcome this long list of sticking points and turn you into a bona fide athlete with the game of *007?*

In this book you'll cover *5 key areas* that when followed consistently will ensure you get in the best shape of your life and Unleash Your Alpha.

You're going to learn to eat like a man should eat, train like an athletic beast, and operate like a true gentleman and become a dead-set legend.

To get the most out of this book, perform the tasks and implement the key take-homes. However, you may wish to read it in its entirety first and come back to each section at a later point.

The 5 key areas include:

1. **Thinking - how thought, desire, and having a mission can unleash your Inner Alpha**

   The way you approach life and each individual day from

within yourself will not only make you a better man, but make life's moments grander and help you tune your A-game. For this to work you must first **choose** to become a better man and lay out the steps to what your life will be and sort your priorities.

2. **Nutrition – you are what you eat: nutrition is king**
   Whether it's fat loss, muscle building, or simply living every day full of energy, what you eat is what your body becomes. You'll discover a framework that breaks nutrition down to a simple guide that saves you time each week.

3. **Training - chiselling the man inside and out**
   Training can be a daunting concept. The programs and framework break this down and make it easy to implement so the man you start seeing in the mirror is that of an eye-catching masculine athlete.

4. **Sleep, stress and enjoyment – the lifestyle of a balanced man**
   How much sleep you get, the quality of it and the amount of unnecessary stress you have play a huge role not only in how you feel during the day, but the state of your body, both inside and out. You'll undertake a process that breaks this down and ensures a fresh man greets each day and makes the most of it.

5. **Man skills – the finer points of being a man**
   For a man to be a true Alpha male, one that knows who he is and lives a life of true masculinity there are certain things that you should "just know." These crucial tips, such as your personal brand, cooking skills, how to act on a date, how

to read your partner, and even how to back a trailer, are the finer points that make a man, and make you an Alpha with an A-game and real control of your life.

This book is exactly that – the perfect step-by-step guide for any man to find their Inner Alpha and become the picture of masculinity.

The above mistakes will look slightly different for everyone, but in the end the common themes ring true. So ask yourself:

Are you making any of the same mistakes?
Is your life going exactly how you'd ~~like it~~, LOVE it to go?

***

Before we kick off, think of your definition of what a man is and what a man should be. Now think of your own characteristics, what people describe you as. How would you describe yourself? Do these match our man, our Alpha?

Now think about what's missing in your life. Are you overweight? Struggle to get laid? Never get the promotion or work you *really* want, constantly living for the weekend and some relative peace until Monday rolls around again? Are you in any way unhappy with your life?

Now close your eyes and imagine that in one year from now none of that's improved – in fact it's worse because of your inaction. Soon you'll be in a hole too big to get out of – stuck in the same job, dealing with the same arseholes every day, but with an even bigger gut.

Now, imagine you look like a ripped athlete with visible abs, you have a life that not only brings home the bacon but makes you *want* to get out of bed in the morning, you have the confidence and game that allowed you to get the partner and relationship of your dreams, or you finally have the drive to actually have sex on a regular basis with your current partner.

Imagine that you have real control in your life, you command respect in any situation and you can get all the sex you want.

And that's one of the keys here – you *want* sex.

Whatever your holes are, imagine them filled and you're now killing it in every aspect of your life. How good would that be?

WHAT IT MEANS TO BE A MAN

REDEFINING ALPHA

"Being male is a matter of birth. Being a man is a matter of age. Being a gentleman is a matter of choice."

– EDWIN LOUIS COLE

Depending on whom you ask, you'll get varying answers on what a man is. The obvious parts are the anatomical and physiological traits, the meat and potatoes. However, what it means to be a man, and what the standard character traits of manhood are is highly contentious. Some that come to mind are *leader, provider, masculine, virile, strong*, yet many would argue that those labels are archaic or obsolete.

In the simplest definition, man is an adult human male. For the most part as our ancestors evolved into early humans, man was the leader, warrior, provider, and father for future generations.

Nowadays, we men have lost our identity. With such variation in what a modern man's roles are, there's considerable confusion. Men are working in every kind of role you can imagine – from traditional roles such as farmers and business leaders to more modern roles like stay-at-home dads.

Whether these differences have caused the trends we're currently seeing or are simply a result of complex changes to society is irrelevant. What's important is that the idea of man, what it means to be a man, and what traits men possess are changing, making us men something we haven't been before – and it's not for the better.

Traditionally a man could easily be summed up by the term *Alpha male*- the *one who led*. However, as we've evolved this term in particular has become lost and misconstrued. It largely carries the negative connotations of a macho arrogant dick. Some good traits used in bad ways.

Let's take a closer look at the term *Alpha Male*.

The Oxford and Collins' dictionary defines *Alpha male* as *the dominant male in a group*. However, these days Alpha is often seen as domineering, macho, arrogant, overzealous, aggressive, and close minded. Of course all these traits can be perfect in certain situations. However, when not balanced with the compassion, integrity, kindness, and caring that our time-honoured Alpha possessed, we often get disaster.

In the corporate world this is very common – men who dominate situations by manipulating others, alienating colleagues, creating fear, expecting the impossible, leaving people feeling demoralised, neglected, unsupported, and bullied.

Studies and surveys in Australia and the US have shown over 33% of employees have suffered some form of bullying, with upwards of 62% of bullies being male.

At home this can and does lead to sexual, physical, and emotional abuse, both spousal and child. The Australian Crime Commission estimates that one in four girls are sexually abused and between one in seven to one in twelve boys experience sexual abuse!

This also affects our social circles and we quite often see an environment of blokey one-up-manship, where men will constantly get into a "my dick is bigger than yours" duel, which leads to the degradation of one man by a more dominant one. All fun and games, until someone gets seriously depressed, doesn't do anything about it for way too long and spirals into an introverted metaphorical man cave, which is deep, dark, and hard to get out of.

It's safe to say that today's description of an Alpha male is far removed from the true Alpha. John Broadbent, author of *Man Unplugged*, and Steve Biddolph, the author of *Raising Boys* and *The New Manhood*, define as:

"Those that know who they are, have 'done the work' on their inner realm and faced their demons, understand that fear is real but not paralysing, and not afraid to challenge the status quo, are in touch with their emotions but not ruled by them, and understand that we have two ears and one mouth and should perhaps use them in that percentage!"

When a man – knows who he is, is confident in his own body, knows how to deal with his emotions, face his fears, can stand resolute when needed, hold his own in conversation, doing so with compassion and integrity – he is showing the true traits of a real Alpha male.

***

Let's call this true modern day Alpha, *Our Alpha*.

We know this guy has backbone, heart, and compassion. He knows when to speak up and he knows when to listen and show empathy and understanding. However, there's much more to being a man than just being a great guy.

What good is a great guy if he's unhealthy? If every man had these Alpha qualities without having real A-game we wouldn't be much further from where we currently are.

So what is A-game? It's that quality a true Alpha has that radiates from him when he enters a room. It's a combination of his appearance, charisma, humility, confidence, and charm. Another crucial part of this is the absence of unnecessary ego. Ego that's obvious and omnipresent is usually making up for some sort of lack in confidence or self-assuredness. Having to prove ego or shove it in the face of others is showing your insecurities and your complete lack of A-game and true Alpha qualities.

According to Elliot D. Cohen PhD, one of the most prevalent fears among men is having a lack of feeling wanted, respected, important and in control. A man with game has these in spades. However, that doesn't *just come* – it's part of a process and combination of qualities that must be honed and worked on.

Ask any man what he *really, truly* wants and most will eventually answer that they want **respect and sex.** It may sound blunt and crass, but it's very true.

Let's look at some characteristics of the Anti-Alpha versus Our Alpha:

Typical Qualities of The Anti-Alpha
- Is a sheep – follows the crowd, or bullies and manipulates others to get his way.
- Doesn't stand up for what he believes in.
- Is happy with being average and mediocre, or is prone to detrimental obsessive behaviours.
- Does what's expected of him and no more.
- Is an awesome time-waster and procrastinator.
- Doesn't know how to stand up for himself or others,

or goes over the top and tries to be "the man," seeking attention.

- Doesn't have goals and desires for the future, or has single-minded and selfish desire without real life perspective.
- Dwells on the past and fears the future.
- Has misplaced priorities and struggles for life perspective.
- Doesn't have too many really strong close relationships.
- Isn't proud of his body, or is arrogant and conceited about his body.
- Has deep-seated confidence issues and low self worth.
- Has a scarcity mindset – thinks others will take his ideas and opportunities.

Typical Qualities of Our Alpha

- Lives his own life.
- Has a set of maxims or rules that he lives by, be they conscious or not.
- Takes pride in his appearance and works on his health, fitness, and body but isn't arrogant.
- Has a subtle confidence and constantly exudes this, without being smug.
- Commands respect and has a strong personal brand that consistently represents him in a great light.
- Knows what drives him and actively seeks it every day, without being fanatical.
- Prioritises the important things in his life and has a balance that allows this.
- Has a positive attitude and outlook on life.
- He has a sense of humour and can laugh at himself.

- Does great things for other people and acts unselfishly often, however, looks after number one when needed.
- Has strong opinions on matters that require it yet still has an open mind.
- Knows that there is more to life than money and material things such as real relationships, which he cherishes and builds.
- Puts in the work to make his life better and the lives of those close to him.
- Isn't afraid to fail and uses failures as learning experiences to grow and improve.
- Doesn't sweat the small stuff and has great perspective in life.
- Goes out of his way to empower and help others and isn't afraid to give his best for free.
- Has an abundance mindset – sees opportunity everywhere.

The A-game we're talking about is a guy who not only has the confidence of an Alpha with his shit sorted, but is in great physical condition. He's the picture of health and masculinity: strong, muscular, lean, and sorted. And his sex drive mirrors that.

A true Alpha with real A-game not only can get laid but he wants to. <=== Tweet that shit! #UnleashYourAlpha @mcampbell2012

This may seem like a backwards point but trust me, when a man has no game it's not just a mental and psychological thing – his body is fighting against him. Hormones are one of the most crucial parts of this puzzle, and one of the most common issues creating the anti-Alpha.

We'll get into the hormones in the next chapter but suffice it to say when your sex drive is lacking, so is your overall game and health. Your hormones can be your best mate or your greatest enemy. Because of the massive effect they have on your body and its reactions, this is going to be an area of focus. We'll outline the issues and give some actionable steps to correct and manage them.

When it comes to painting this picture of our Alpha, talking to those who seek out men and are attracted to men – namely women and gay men – provides enlightening opinion. The overwhelming reaction when asked about the state of men is usually like an emphatic, "Hell yes, where are all the *real* men?"

One such example is someone I interviewed for this book, Andrew Creagh, the editor and founder of Australia's biggest gay men's magazine and a gay man himself. He has an amazing insight being both as a man and someone attracted to men.

He brought up a brilliant present day example: Russian president Vladimir Putin draws on what we would call very old-fashioned ideas of masculinity to bolster his popularity. He goes bareback horse riding, scuba diving and brings up lost treasure, practises judo, flies a hang glider that leads a flock of lost geese home. There's even an action comic book starring Putin that's sold to kids.

It's all carefully micromanaged by his PR team but it obviously resonates with Russians. He's painting himself as Alpha, however, he's clearly falling into the macho anti-Alpha – do real men have PR teams to take care of their actions? No, because if there's one thing a real man should be it's authentic! That kind of behaviour is definitely not authentic.

Andrew also points out a comparison: look at Henry Fonda's role in the movie *12 Angry Men*. He plays the smart, philosopher type whose intellect finally wins out against the loud, physically aggressive bully. He's the only juror who believes an accused murderer should be acquitted because of reasonable doubt. His masculinity is standing by his beliefs in the face of adversity or overwhelming opposition. He's showing the traits of a true Alpha.

Celebrity chef Pete Evans, has a brilliant description that I think suits as we leave this chapter:

"To be an alpha is just to be you. Don't copy someone else. Take inspiration, but you know what's right for you. You know when you're being fake, it shows as a weakness because it's insecurity. I think the most powerful people in the world are the ones that are very confident in themselves.

Being a man is a package.

Everyone loves to do something, but people have so many excuses why they can't do it- success is waking up with a smile on your face."

The Alpha we aspire to be is a strong, confident, healthy man. Has control in his life, knows who he is and what he wants. He looks great and feels even better. He's a man who others simply want to be around.

"The ancient Greeks understood this positive male energy, calling it 'Zeus Energy' – which encompasses intelligence, robust health, compassionate decisiveness, good will, generous leadership. Zeus energy is male authority accepted for the sake of the community."

ROBERT BLY IN *IRON JOHN*

THE PROBLEMS

WHAT'S GONE SO WRONG?

"...We're just walking around, looking around. We like women, we want women, but that's pretty much as far as we've got. That's why we're honking car horns, yelling from construction sites- we're working on some new programs, but it's not easy when your mind's a blank.

Why do men do these things? Why do men behave so badly?

Men are not developing, we're not improving. We men know that no matter how poorly we behave, it seems we somehow end up with women anyway. Look around, beautiful women, men are with them. Do you think these are special men, gifted highly unusual, one of a kind men? These are the same jerks and idiots I'm talking about"

– JERRY SEINFELD

We men have bigger waistlines than ever, soaring rates of disease and worrying statistics for divorce, job satisfaction, depression, and suicide.

Let's look at exactly what is happening to us men and why it's happening.

The main issues we face are:

1. Being de-conditioned – hormonally screwed, leading to being overweight, unfit, weak, inflexible, poor posture, poor sleep patterns, various illness, and diseases.

2. Low self-confidence and self worth.
3. Undersexed, either due to low sex drive or simply not getting as much as we'd like.

Why is this happening?

Why are we carrying too much body fat and not enough muscle mass? Why are we constantly faced with nagging injuries and illness? Why are we unhealthy and de-conditioned? Why do we have low self worth? Why is depression and general dissatisfaction with life so rampant? Why are we not enjoying a great and healthy sex life?

We're in bad shape. For the most part we're simply eating the wrong foods, not doing enough exercise or the right kind, live over stressed lives, don't get enough quality sleep and have our priorities all mixed up.

These elements work as a whole and when one or more is affected then so are the other elements, leading to a sense of unbalance. Left unchecked, this unbalance can and *will* present itself as a physical, emotional and/or spiritual dysfunction.

Here's a typical scenario:

You're spending too much time at work and not enough quality time doing things you enjoy. This starts to cause higher levels of stress, which is usually handled very poorly and encroaches on the time you do get away from work. Sleep suffers dramatically and this vicious cycle becomes a downward spiral.

This can result in losing respect at home and any real control in your life. Fear can start to take over as a dominant motivator of our actions – the fear of losing respect at home, in our social situations, and in our work environment become huge. A fear of rejection from partners or potential partners is also a real prospect.

This all leads to a perceived loss of control which in turn leads to an actual real loss of control. Not great for us men when we want to be in charge of our lives and dominating our days.

From here if we decide to make a positive change and start getting in better shape there's so much information out there it becomes similar to being dropped at sea. It's confusing, overwhelming, and often conflicting.

All this does to us men is act as a metaphorical kick in the balls when we finally wanted to improve ourselves. The confidence weans further and we're back into our downward spiral. Now the weight keeps piling on, the confidence continues to drop, you struggle to emotionally or intelligently articulate this to yourself let alone others and soon you haven't had sex in months and you're getting depressed.

Let's hear the thoughts on this from an expert; Dr Phillips, whose special expertise and particular interest is in depressive disorders as well as forensic psychiatry:

"A lot of men feel they are inadequate and fear how they can get on in the world, and that's really about survival and, when you start talking to them, their level of esteem is far less than it ought to be. It's hard to build the esteem and build the sense of comfort with self and comfort with others. We do live in a pretty mercenary society and the quest for possessions and property is way over valued when really we should be looking at happiness and contentment."

Paleoanthropologist Peter McAlister in his book *Manthropology* discusses the state of present day man and how as a whole we're the weakest we've ever been. Not just compared to some of our early hominid brothers such as the Neanderthals from more than 1 million years ago, but when compared to early humans, even as close as the ancient Greeks or Genghis Kahn and his posse of warriors.

McAlister and his colleagues have used various techniques to show that the average male skeleton throughout different periods in history before ours was thicker and had more healed abrasions and major injuries – meaning that these men had more muscle mass and greater capacity to take a decent knock and then get back to health and continue being a provider.

This is alarming when compared to the relatively soft men we see in abundance today. This isn't to say every man has to be a tough as nails Neaderthal-esque brute, but that an ingrained toughness which sees a more common masculine physique and steadfastness to withstand life's little knockbacks is seriously missing today when compared to men throughout history.

It's also not to say that every man who is strong and in great shape is a true Alpha. There are ripped arseholes everywhere – this is not a well-rounded man. However, to unleash your Alpha you must be mentally *and* physically strong.

Why this stuff happens is sometimes a chicken and egg situation. Are we overweight because we eat poorly or do we eat poorly because we're overweight and can't find the time, motivation, or energy to do anything about it?

Are we unhealthy because we have too much stress and not enough quality sleep or are we tired and stressed because we're unhealthy, out of shape, and are constantly busy?

When it comes to gaining weight everyone seems to *know* what the cause is – too much food and not enough exercise. This is a far too simplistic way to look at it. Gains in body fat result from more than just eating too much and not exercising enough – our bodies are very complicated organisms, and simple thermodynamics of energy-in versus energy-out just doesn't cut it. To leave it there would be doing everyone reading this a gross injustice.

One of the main factors that affect what your body looks like and how you feel every day is what your hormones are doing in response to *all* of your lifestyle factors.

WHERE THE PROBLEMS LIE

"There is no more male idea in the history of the universe than why don't we fly up to the moon and drive around?"

– JERRY SEINFELD

How many men do you know that second-guess themselves on a daily basis? Sentences like, "Yeah I dunno honey, whatever you want." are commonplace from a guy who is essentially being dominated by his partner because he has no gumption to take lead of a situation and own it.

How many men rave about how happy their lives are? The media doesn't help, but so many men are in a long-standing rut, doing the same thing every day, no real satisfaction and only intermittent happiness.

What about a sentence like, "Yeah I've been slowly packing on the pounds since I've been office bound," or "I sleep poorly and my energy through the day hits big slumps mid morning and mid afternoon?" Both of these are incredibly common.

It needn't be this way.

The current rate of obesity in men worldwide is astonishing and growing by the day. In Australia alone the rate of overweight and obese men was at 70% according to *The Australian Bureau Of Statistics* for 2011-2012, with 42% of men overweight and 28% obese.

Let me break that down – for every 100 guys that read this book, on average, 70 of you will be overweight or obese! That's just the tip of the iceberg when it comes to problems relating to it. That compares to a relative 56% for women.

We're doing something wrong fellas.

Obesity leads to a myriad of diseases and conditions such as type II diabetes, cardiovascular disease, chronic joint pain, and depression just to name a few.

One of the biggest issues we have is an absence of foresight into what all these little issues will become if left unchanged and what to do about it if there is any recognition. Another is ego. This is a case where ignorance isn't bliss, as it's leading you to the raft of conditions our anti-Alpha faces.

Ego creates a false alpha of macho bravado. We tell ourselves *"I'll be alright,"* rather than admitting to even the most serious health problems.

This lack of awareness and complete ignorance is sending today's men on an unpleasant journey to an early grave. This also comes with a lack of true confidence and standing on your own two feet.

This can lead to long-term unhappiness and depression as well as some of these more common consequences like obesity, diabetes, heart conditions, and loss of fertility and sex drive.

According to John Broadbent, author of *Man...Unplugged,* one of the most common things he sees when working with men is this lack of real conviction to stand strong with your opinions, an inability to make your feelings known, let alone get them across and the eventual tactic to, "suffer in silence."

John and some of his contemporaries have done a lot of work and research into certain causes of this eventual downward spiral of men today and the things that most seem to agree on is that during our upbringing we have lost the rite of passage that was once a normal part of society.

We fail to develop our identity and a real sense of worth from our fathers, and this has led to boys and girls being raised the same way. *New York Times* best-selling author Marianne Williamson said, "We created a generation of hard women and soft men." This is reflected in the isolation dislocation – deep inner man-cave – that we see in men today along with soaring rates of depression and suicide.

People who suffer from mental illness also suffer from every other major illness in much larger numbers, making getting on top of mental health a real priority.

Dr Jonathan Phillips' take on depression is fascinating, and *worrying*:

> *"We know that one in five Australian men, woman and children in any given year have a diagnosable mental health disorder. And very few of them in fact know and even fewer get assessed. Very few of them will do anything about it. And the trick with mental health problems is intervention at an early time.*
>
> *Depression is probably the illness, which causes the greatest health burden worldwide at the present time. And the thing to keep in mind with depression and for anxiety is that it's very common. It's eminently treatable and the trick is early intervention, be it intervention by way of a coach or a mentor or specialist."*

The statistics alone are a huge worry. When we look at what else results from this struggle for men to speak their mind, own their own space and deal with their emotions in a healthy and normal manner. We see alcoholism increase as well as rates of domestic violence and abuse. The number of children assaulted and sexually abused is on the rise. During the period 2005-2010 abuse and assault by family members and known non-family members all rose significantly.

In her book *He'll Be Ok*, Celia Lashlie wrote that during her time as a prison warden in New Zealand she saw young Maori males in particular use prison as a rite of passage as they weren't getting this through normal societal means. Their rite of passage is *doing time*.

It's this rite of passage that seems to be absent in today's society for young men. According to Steve Biddulph in his book *The New Manhood*, if you get 100 men in a room, 30 of them don't talk to their dads, *ever* – completely estranged. Thirty of them connect for Christmas and Birthdays, 30 of them have some sort of relationship, where they can go to footy and have a sort of conversation. But only 10 actually have what he would call a functional relationship with their dads.

This has never been like this before throughout history. Traditionally you'd be with your father as you grew up out in the farm, in the mill, or whatever he did and he would give you tasks appropriate to your age to help you mature through that process.

Now boys are being raised increasingly by women, taught by women, and we're missing this crucial rite of passage. According to John Broadbent the most common theme he's seen in young males is this simmering rage. These males are lost, they don't really know who they are, where they've come from or where they belong and without this rite of passage and proper masculine modelling they go looking for it elsewhere.

Steve Biddulph said, "If you don't teach a boy how to find their compass, they'll be drawn by other people's magnetic fields and they'll travel through life lost." This was reinforced by Broadbent who states that, "Because of the lack of mentoring that we've had through lack of fathering, lack of male figures, lack of role models, lack of male school teachers a lot of boys grow up into men without a compass. They've got no idea which direction they're going. They just stumble from disaster to disaster. And these may be CEO's and business leaders."

Just look at the kind of "role models" we see everyday – Tiger Woods, Lance Armstrong, Charlie Sheen – all legends and successes in their own right, but in terms of being appropriate role models for young males, they've got *massive* flaws that will send boys into macho, arrogant anti-Alphas.

This is an example of a real role model; I asked celebrity chef and father of two young girls, Pete Evans, how he approaches being a role model to his kids, and he explained the aspects of a masculine role model very succinctly:

"For me a masculine role model is about being in the best possible emotional, physical and mental shape; the whole thing. So that whenever my girls associate their father or a masculine figure, they feel safe around them. Around me. It's about teaching my kids that they can do anything and don't have to go with the crowd. It's about understanding what the difference is between right and wrong. I think you need to be present, listen and you need to engage and have fun on all levels. If you can look at it through their eyes as much as yours, I think that's the key. We all make mistakes and get caught up in our own shit. I think you just need a gentle reminder everyday that this is what life is about."

I love this description as it nails the point which we sadly don't see enough of at the moment. Without this traditional or normal rite of passage from functioning and appropriate male role models we're developing a generation of dysfunctional youths that are only going to exacerbate the current state of anti-Alphas quickly spreading throughout society.

Largely today, men have gone from the figure of provider and protector to suspicious being. This was summed up brilliantly by Sir Bob Geldolf:

"We've demonised men. Men really are sort of considered brutish and hairy, and unemotional, and aggressive, and loud, and smelly ... and this big hairy thing between their legs. That is seriously present in a lot of current thinking. This is a disgrace. This truly is a disgrace, where you view a man as a suspicious being. Men, in general, are a protector. We have seen a complete perversity, a complete change of what men are, and what they're supposed to be. We've almost lost our reason with regard to it."

***

We also see a large shift in the collective energies in society. Every person, male and female will have elements of masculine energy and feminine energy. Ideally a man will have stronger masculine energy but still be in touch with his feminine energy and know that part of him, and the reverse for females.

However, with the much needed rise of women, equality and feminism over the last 50 years, we've allowed the oppression of our masculinity and the feminine has started to become the dominant energy. This is why we see such an abundance of men with low confidence and self worth.

Now in order for this to balance out, women have had to pick up the slack and take over the dominant masculine energy space.

In his book *The Way Of The Superior Man*, David Deida points out that we've reached "a 50/50 intermediate stage of growth, which sees economic and social equality, but sexual neutrality – bank accounts are balancing while passion is fizzing out".

So instead of the two opposing energies working in perfect unison, we have a neutral meeting in the middle, causing the society we see today – weak men with a lack of identity, overtly macho or overtly wimpy – and strong women with a lack of understanding about the men in their lives. This vicious cycle is only spiralling further down the longer it goes on.

There's absolutely nothing wrong with a guy knowing and owning his feminine qualities, it's being owned by them that's the issue.

Dr Jonathan Phillips also has an important point when it comes to these two sides of every man:

"Freud talked about the animus and the anima. The male animus that runs inside all people and the female anima. And there's some balance there. A well-rounded person carries both within him or her. Obviously in man there's going to be more on one side than the other. But it is the balance. And I think one of the important things for an Alpha male in fact, is to be aware of his sensitivities, the need to have empathy and to understand and be able to get close to others. It's finding a balance. It's not one or the other, it's finding a balance; be in touch with ones emotions, have a good understanding of them, be comfortable with them but not having the emotions dominate the man."

Again, another clear and distinct definition of a true Alpha – in touch with but not ruled by his emotions and feminine side.

All these issues mean hormones are affected greatly, and a massive drop in sex drive and fertility occurs – two of the main indicators of masculine health. At a basic biological and evolutionary level we live in order to procreate and continue the survival of the species and in particular your bloodline.

If this most basic and primal of male attributes is missing or lacking then we have already lost our way as men and our part in this world. However, with modern medicine's ability to control so many conditions and diseases, the anti-Alpha continues to expand his bloodline despite a non-existent sex drive and the fertility that a giant panda would be ashamed of.

It's not necessarily just our complex hormonal system that causes this. Many men who don't have any say in their relationship – they don't wear, or more accurately, *share* the pants – witness a drop in their sex drive because they simply *aren't allowed* to have sex very often. This problem increases as they let it happen repeatedly.

Without playing their part as true Alpha male and having some say and control in situations such as these, the anti-Alpha loses confidence further, goes deep into his inner man-cave, never speaks up and the example mentioned earlier regarding relationships breaking up becomes a real and sad threat.

How many times have you heard a married man complain about his lack of sex and lack of satisfaction? Not a recipe for a happy man.

***

Look at your life from the outside. Are you making any of these mistakes or suffering from any of these issues? Be truthful and open to change, because that acceptance and willingness to change will help you grow and become a better man.

Let's start that process and figure out what it is that's going on in your body (and mind).

A BIT OF SCIENCE –
DONE SIMPLY

"Everything must be made as simple as possible. But not simpler."

ALBERT EINSTEIN

Hormones can be a frightening word when we don't know much about them. We frequently go straight to thoughts of females and their "time of the month." However, that's where we're largely just uninformed.

As men, things such as how much gut you see sticking out when you take a piss, what your quality of sleep is like, how your body reacts to the food you eat and whether you want to or can have sex are fuelled by and rely on our complex hormonal processes.

You've most likely heard of insulin, testosterone, and estrogen, but what about human growth hormone, cortisol, leptin, ghrelin and glucagon? Many of our body's basic functions work according to these key hormones. One of the main key functions is our *metabolism*.

When it comes to regulating metabolic rate and metabolism, these hormones all play different parts, but to approach fat loss or muscle gain without considering these is equivalent to learning to drive a car blindfolded - you might get somewhere but it won't be very far in the direction you desire. Cortisol also plays a huge part in our body's response to stressors and how we sleep. Leptin and ghrelin affect appetite regulation as well as work to maintain relative energy equilibrium.

Whether extra fat is causing high estrogen or vice versa isn't our focus right now, we simply want to know what these hormones do and what we want to promote.

In short, our hormones are a complex series of inter-related functions that work together globally and therefore must be looked at in that way. From now on your hormones are going to be one of your biggest weapons. We want to optimize as much as possible.

Some of these hormones are *Anabolic,* which means that they promote growth; while some are *Catabolic* meaning they break down bigger molecules into smaller ones.

So let's get catabolic with our words and break these hormones down (*Side note – dad jokes allowed, they just must be clever, like this one…*):

Insulin – Insulin is a hugely important part of your normal day-to-day functioning. Insulin's main role is to regulate blood sugar or blood glucose. It's secreted from the pancreas in response to carbohydrates entering the blood stream and becoming blood glucose. Insulin's job is to help the body process this glucose by binding to receptors on your cells to absorb the glucose from your blood stream into the cell to be used as energy.

It also acts to facilitate the uptake of muscle building amino acids into the cells so our muscles can grow. This is crucial in our post-workout window. What this means is if you eat foods that manage insulin secretion or your body is sensitive to insulin it runs like a well oiled machine; the insulin pulls the glucose into the cells for use as energy or stores it in the muscles as glycogen to be used at another time.

However, if your body is insulin resistant, the glucose doesn't absorb into the cells and you're left with increased glucose in your blood, requiring further insulin be secreted from your pancreas to try to deal with this. This leads to the increased glucose in the blood stream, which is stored as body fat.

Let's look at it in a way that might be easier to understand – think of insulin as the bouncer to the club. If *insulin sensitive,* the bouncer opens the door and the glucose moves on through to party. If *insulin resistant* the bouncer doesn't have glucose on the guest list. No glucose gets into the club so it stays out in the hot street that is your blood stream.

The boss of the club, your pancreas, thinks more bouncers are needed to deal with all the glucose outside so it releases more. Now you've got loads of bouncers and club goers out in the street but neither going where they should. The club is empty and void of the energetic partygoer glucose it needs to operate optimally. This leads to a rocket fuel in the blood stream of too much glucose and insulin, resulting in a myriad of negative effects including increased fat storage and risk of critical diseases.

The good news is these terms *insulin resistance* and *insulin sensitivity* aren't rigid and respond to certain lifestyle factors from what you eat to what training you do. We're going to address your nutrition in a later chapter, but your take home point is: **Many men have trouble regulating insulin, with insulin resistance a common problem. We want to promote good management of insulin and its positive anabolic response through a variety of lifestyle factors including diet, training, and stress management to get and keep you lean, ripped, and healthy – key attributes of our Alpha.**

Glucagon – This distant planet-sounding hormone works in opposition and balance to insulin, so we must get a quick grasp on what it does and why it's important. Just as insulin works to lower blood glucose levels by diffusing through the cell wall, glucagon acts to release glucose into the blood when levels are too low. It's released from the pancreas and mostly stimulates the liver to convert some of its stored glycogen into glucose so your blood has some energy for you to function.

It also acts to stimulate lipolysis, which is the mobilization of fat mass to create free fatty acids also to be used as fuel. As this is a releasing or stimulating hormone, compared to insulin's storage nature, it acts to get the body moving and therefore increase metabolism. So while excess insulin leads to your body storing energy and converting excess glucose to fat, glucagon will act to speed up your body's ability to use fuel.

So using our example from above, your blood stream is low on party goers (glucose), so the club boss (your pancreas) holds a promotion in conjunction with your liver to get more party goers out in the street so they can eventually make their way into the club (the cell) so a party can take place i.e., energy burned in order to keep the status quo or homeostasis.

Take home point: insulin and glucagon work in contrast to each other, but always in an attempt to reach a relative cellular and blood equilibrium. For us to get the positive effects of insulin we need to maximise this relationship.

Testosterone – Much more than a by-product of a bunch of men talking about women, sports, and generally being competitive and chauvinistic, testosterone is one of your main anabolic hormones. It's crucial not only for growth of muscle, connective tissue, and bone but also your overall health and well being.

Testosterone is our man hormone – it's the big daddy that so many men are low in today and that needs to be addressed to turn our plight around. Testosterone's anabolic nature promotes protein synthesis and the growth of tissue. Proteins are the building blocks of our body; so to promote protein synthesis we are promoting growth.

With testosterone production causing an increase in this protein synthesis we're seeing an environment that's conducive to the growth of new tissue and of particular relevance, new muscle. For us this is a good environment and one we want to endorse. More muscle mass will result in an increase in metabolism which will in turn make you a fat burning machine.

However, testosterone is also responsible for the one function we kind of know about already – male sexual arousal – and is key for normal sperm development and determining your sex drive. An easy relationship to make is that if you have a low sex drive, one of the culprits to look at is your testosterone and vice versa. If you're a horny bastard there's a good chance your testosterone could be looking okay. This doesn't mean you're Alpha; just that you may have okay T levels.

In men, testosterone is produced in our testes and in response to certain stimuli this will fluctuate. Testosterone works in direct relation to the catabolic hormone cortisol to promote protein synthesis while inhibiting the catabolic effects of hard training. This is known as your testosterone-to-cortisol ratio.

As we saw above, high levels of blood glucose and insulin will inhibit testosterone, as will poor sleep and high stress levels. Low stress levels, quality deep sleep, effective nutrition and training all help to promote its release and proper functioning. Easy to see how this stuff is all interrelated, right?

It's been shown that men with higher levels of testosterone are less likely to have high blood pressure, suffer from heart attacks, and be obese.

Conversely, low testosterone levels have been shown to be associated with increased risk of type II diabetes, cancer (in particular prostate cancer) as well as decreased bone density, muscle mass and strength, and increased risk and incidence of depression.

Take home point: Many men have undiagnosed low testosterone. We want to promote testosterone production to have an optimal hormonal balance and to encourage muscle building, strong bones and joints, fat loss, a healthy heart, and a sex drive Ron Jeremy would be proud of. All key attributes of our Alpha.

Human growth hormone (HGH) – HGH is another vital anabolic hormone responsible for promoting growth, as the name suggests, tissue repair, and regeneration. HGH is released from the pituitary gland in bursts throughout the day in response to different stimuli including the food you eat, what training you do, your sleep, stress, and other hormonal activity as a part of our complex global endocrine system.

HGH stimulates the repair and regeneration of tissue including bone, connective tissue and muscle. One of its main functions is to manage body fat and lean mass by boosting protein synthesis and the creation of new muscle. HGH also acts to stimulate the breakdown of fat mass to be used as fuel (lipolysis).

Now here's the kicker for those of you who think sleep isn't that important – HGH levels are highest during deep sleep and secretion occurs in waves throughout our sleep. If we have poor sleep and this HGH cycle and production is interrupted then you'll suffer with low and inconsistent levels. So getting a good night sleep is crucial to optimise HGH levels and all the benefits that come with it.

Take home point: we want to encourage optimal HGH levels

to aid the anabolic activities of protein synthesis and muscle repair while keeping you lean and strong.

Estrogen – Sometimes the culprit and scapegoat for our women folk, estrogen is the primary *female* sex hormone. However, that mustn't be mistaken for *female only* hormones, as estrogens are present in males too, as well as in our environment.

Like testosterone, estrogens are steroid hormones, meaning they pass through the cell membrane easily and once inside the cell act to bind with estrogen receptors, which is when they can start to play a huge role in your body. In men, estrogen acts to regulate certain roles of the reproductive system and plays a part in the maturation of sperm.

Alongside testosterone, estrogen forms a ratio that we naturally sit at. If this ratio moves towards estrogen then we start to see all kinds of negative effects on your body including sexual characteristics.

Estrogens also come from the environment as things such as plastic water bottles, skin care, and cosmetics such as moisturisers and sunscreen, even things like credit card transaction receipts. These environmental estrogens can join forces with the estrogen inside you and have many negative effects such as increased fat storage, loss of muscle mass, infertility, and fat storage in more "female" areas such as the hips and formation of breasts aka "man boobs", or "moobs."

We can also see erectile dysfunction, depression, and a decrease in the positive effect testosterone has due to it's low levels.

These effects, in particular fat gain and high insulin all act to increase aromatase, an enzyme that works to synthesize androgens. This means testosterone gets synthesized into more estrogen, leading to more of the negative effects mentioned above. So it goes, until you're faced with your own moobs and child-bearing hips, little or decreasing muscle mass, very low sex drive, and a fertility issue.

Take home point: we want to ensure optimal estrogen levels by avoiding unnecessary environmental sources and keeping your body's levels at a healthy balance with testosterone. This comes down to lifestyle factors including sleep, training, nutrition, and alcohol consumption.

Cortisol – Produced from cholesterol and released from our adrenal glands in response to stress, cortisol's effects are many and varied in your body's constant struggle to maintain homeostasis, or relative normality.

One of cortisol's main roles is as a response to a "fight or flight" stimulus. Another hormone, adrenaline (or epinephrine) also acts in this fight or flight response to mobilise stored energy to be used as fuel in a very primal survival response.

The mechanism at work is to supply a boost of energy by way of a release of glucose into the blood stream to either fight or leave in a hurry. This is done at the expense of other bodily functions to prioritize survival.

Due to this process, cortisol's role is also to hinder or essentially block insulin from doing its job – in this stressful situation your body wants extra glucose pumping around the body, not being stored for future considerations.

However, this means high levels of cortisol will lead to high levels of glucose in the blood – high blood glucose – not a good thing in the long run, with insulin being halted from doing its job, all this cortisol and glucose in the blood means insulin resistance becomes a real threat.

Now your poor old pancreas can't keep up with all this glucose and soon increased fat mass, lean mass breakdown, and risk of chronic diseases such as diabetes and heart disease becomes a major problem.

Next, cortisol also has more key roles that affect us greatly on a daily basis. Inflammation is generally something we want to avoid and deal with as efficiently as possible. Certain lifestyle factors such as a bad diet and high levels of stress will elevate inflammatory levels.

Cortisol is released to fight this inflammation and restore this relative normal, however, it's also responsible for suppressing the immune system in doing do. So when we see chronic inflammation from a constant assault of stressors and poor lifestyle choices, we see our immune system relentlessly suppressed and becoming a shadow of what our Alpha's immune system looks like.

Furthermore, cortisol also activates your sympathetic nervous system, which acts to respond in the situations described above (fight or flight) and with this active our parasympathetic nervous system becomes dormant.

At certain times this is vital as this system is designed for "rest and repair." It not only helps us recover, it's crucial to properly digest our foods by allowing the enzymes and hormones that control digestion to do their job and absorb the nutrients for use.

Now think about what would happen if you eat when you're stressed, inflamed, and pumping with cortisol – your gut will suffer, your digestion and absorption are affected.

Threat of indigestion is like a pirate ship waiting to board a weakened vessel while still barraging it with cannons of cortisol – soon your gut becomes inflamed and damaged, leading to more cortisol and more of the same.

However, the *acute* affect of cortisol is crucial for our health and survival. Unlike the anabolic, or growth promoting hormones discussed already, this is a catabolic hormone that acts to break down tissue, including the breakdown of triglycerides into free fatty acids to be used as fuel.

Without this response to things such as hard training we couldn't benefit from the subsequent anabolic response of hormones like testosterone and HGH. However, it's *chronic* high levels of cortisol that are of huge concern and incredibly common in men today.

Take home point: Poor lifestyle choices including bad diet, incorrect training, high levels of stress, and constant worry can cause cortisol to flourish at high levels. This can lead to poor gut health, insulin resistance, and a weakened immune system. Following the right training, nutrition, and lifestyle, cortisol can be used to optimise the global hormonal activity and where you sit on our Alpha continuum.

Leptin & Ghrelin – For most day-to-day functioning your body wants to maintain a level of homeostasis. That's where these two hormones come into play. Ghrelin acts to tell your body that it's hungry while leptin informs your body that it's full.

Ghrelin is produced in the stomach and sends a message to your brain telling you to eat while leptin is secreted in fat cells in response to different stimuli. It generally occurs in the body in direct relation to how much body fat you have – the more fat you have the higher leptin will be.

The primary role of leptin is to determine your level of fullness (satiety) when eating, however, what it's essentially controlling is your energy balance. So not only will it say, "Hey brain, in case you hadn't noticed, your stomach is full! Who put you in charge?" It will also talk to your brain to control energy expenditure to maintain energy equilibrium.

So if we have higher levels of leptin the brain is getting signals of fullness and too much food. What it attempts to do to counter this is burn energy through an increase in metabolism and fat oxidation, as well as the aforementioned appetite control.

But if your levels of leptin get low, such as with extreme dieting, your body acts to counter its effects and restore balance. It will *decrease* metabolism and fat oxidation in order to hold on to fat, while causing an *increase in appetite,* which can in turn lead to a further gain in fat mass.

As leptin is synthesised in the fat cells, this results in the body holding onto fat to survive, as it thinks it's in a state of famine. 'Dieting' and poor food choices, as well as other lifestyle factors that lead to weight gain will in turn lead to *extra* weight gain through these mechanisms of leptin.

When we start to store and continuously hold excess body fat, leptin levels will increase to try to tell your body to stop and burn some energy stores. However, a constant barrage of poor lifestyle choices that promote fat gain results in your body becoming *resistant* to leptin in much the same way it does to insulin, as we spoke about earlier. The storage of fat is once again promoted.

This is how someone can appear to be thin, but actually have high body fat percentage.

Starting to see how this cocktail works as a cycle thats' dependent on the choices you make every day?

As we can see, manipulating leptin and ghrelin can have major roles in our body composition and our overall health and well being.

Take home point: Controlling your hunger is more than just your mind. Your food choices in conjunction with other key lifestyle factors play an integral part in managing these two important hormones. This determines what role they play in your global network of hormonal activity that controls your body composition and you as an Alpha.

From the above summaries we can see that our hormones are essential – they work in all sorts of ways, depending on many factors that we often take for granted in our everyday lives.

We can also see that many problems we face are due to, and in direct relation to hormones, often in combination of many. Our bodies are very intelligent organisms, making them complicated at the best of times.

So when we look at why we're overweight, why we're struggling to manage our energy levels or why we're struggling with any confidence within ourselves, we must consider this complex system and the intricacies of our body and its hormones. It's not called the endocrine *system* for nothing.

So to fill the hole that is missing in your life, whether it be putting on some previously non-existent muscle, dropping the "spare tyre," rediscovering your sex drive or just getting a decent night's sleep for once and feeling healthy, energetic and confident; we absolutely must take an approach that considers all the relevant factors at play.

We must understand that carrying some extra fat will affect our confidence from more than just the psychological disdain for carrying the kilos, but also that your hormones are fighting against you.

One of the main contributors to these problems is pride, stubbornness, and ego. Many guys won't act or ask for help until rock bottom hits and there truly is no other option. To equate it to a few common ailments:

- Nagging pains and small injuries when left become serious and debilitating injuries.
- Low energy and confidence means never reaching any sort of potential or *real* happiness.
- The odd bit of extra weight becomes a large gut, obesity, and chronic disease.

- Slightly off blood work and hormonal profiles become disease and endless prescription medication.
- A gradual loss of strength becomes a weak, brittle skeleton, bone breaks, osteoarthritis and joint replacements.
- Unhappy feelings become full on depression and a complete withdrawal into "the man cave."

It doesn't have to be this way.

There are solutions and it's okay to put yourself first, look after the boss, and take charge of your life, health, and future. In fact, **I implore you to!**

You're going to go through an approach in this book that will break down these key lifestyle areas and give you the information and tools to master this complex system that is your body and everything inside it.

THE SOLUTIONS

HOW TO UNLEASH YOUR ALPHA

"Sometimes the questions are complicated and the answers are simple."

– DR. SEUSS

The solutions to these many problems don't have to be confusing. They're not easy, mind you, but easy to understand and implement.

Let's get you on track and following the uncomplicated plan that not only works for me but that I've seen work for many men before you. This plan is going to be comprehensive *and* simple, it's going to cover many aspects of your life and it's going to turn you into an athlete, a legend, and an Alpha. All areas must be covered to start living a life that you truly love.

Pete Evans put it so well when I asked him about his approach to living an awesome life:

"I'm nearly 40 and I've started really looking after my health over the last two years and I look at photos of myself a couple of years ago and I thought I was looking good, I look better now. And that's not from an ego point; I thought- wow what a transformation can happen in a short period of time from just changing a few habits or

ideas. I can't wait to see what I've done by the time I'm 50.
That excites me. It doesn't scare me looking to the future."

An all over approach to life – starting with mindfulness and happiness, knowing yourself and doing things that make *you* happy – is where we'll kick off.

We've had a very brief look at what our solutions are earlier on. Now it's time to get more depth and flesh out what they involve and how you're going to implement these steps to unleash you inner Alpha, find your A-game and become a legend in your own right.

***

There's no quick fix, no "7-minute abs" – it requires a plan, consistency, and hard work on many areas.

I've created, refined, and constantly improved my system. I've seen it work on countless men and I know the amazingly positive effects it can have physically, mentally, and emotionally.

However, having already seen that one of the major problems is our hormones and mental health, here's the opinion of a leader in the field. Dr Phillips shares his general approach to creating better mental health, fighting depression and mental illness:

"If it is going to bring about real change in people it has to
be holistic. Anything less than attending to the whole is
ultimately inadequate. Sleep, hygiene, exercise, nutrition,
are all part of the package.

Looking towards the goals of life, looking towards how
one will get there, looking at the mistakes that one makes
and how best to rectify them.

Be aware of himself number one. Be prepared to listen
to those who he respects and loves and be prepared to

put effort into bringing about positive change.

Being aware and wanting to do something to improve the situation, and looking after one's self- covering relationships, nutrition, fitness and spiritual life, that being religious or not.

I think coaching or mentoring is good because some people just can't do it themselves. For whatever reason, if it brings existential peace and a sense of security and a sense of mastering the world and contentment, then surely that's a good thing. And indeed if you achieve all of those things, important point, all indicators of health improve- physical and mental."

YOUR FIRST TASKS

Before you start reading the following pages, we're going to work on some of your habits. Creating and cementing behavioural change is priority number one*:*

Convince: Write a letter to yourself as if you were applying for this and you had to convince yourself (and me) you needed to get into the program. Detail where you life is at, what you'd like to improve and where you'd like it to go. Rank yourself in a variety of areas (see your downloadable bonus material for a guide on this unleashyouralpha.com/book-bonus-materials).

Move: Regardless of what you currently do, this week make sure you move, with at least moderate intensity, **4 times.** That's 4 workouts. Look at your week, plan, make time and execute.

Hydrate: Make sure you're drinking roughly at least 2 litres of water. We'll start addressing this in more detail later, but for now, get hydrating throughout the day!

Remove the crap: Go to your kitchen and remove/throw out any obviously shitty food. For this stuff to get removed from your diet you need to remove it from your house, otherwise, it'll get eaten – *remove now!*

Record: Start keeping track of everything you eat and drink. Make sure you're completely honest; this is for you and you only. Also note your energy throughout each day and how you sleep.

Measure: We're not going to be jumping on the scales every day, but you need to capture the start of your journey. Take photos – front, side & back – and take measurements of your chest, waist, hips, thighs, and arms.

Eliminate: For the next 12 weeks you need to eliminate booze as much as possible. That isn't to say you can't introduce the odd beer, vino, or scotch back in later on, but for now to get to Alpha status you have to sacrifice a little to find and earn your balance.

***

One of the biggest limiting factors to making and implementing the necessary changes laid out here is *time*. People love to use time as an excuse for why they can't or haven't changed.

From now on you must not. Time management is going to be crucial, but so is getting your priorities sorted to match what you *really* want – this you'll be finding out shortly.

To offer some perspective on time management and priorities, let's hear from Managing Director of global fitness company

Fitness First, Pete Manuel. Pete has had a remarkable career, spanning four countries and high level positions in companies like *Duracell, Gillette,* and *Procter & Gamble* before joining *Fitness First* as CEO. This is a man who has had an incredible demand on his time yet who came into the fitness industry with some long established habits and routines around health and exercise:

> *"For most people I think it's not always finding the balance between work and family. I think they're in a position where they're not always making choices to benefit themselves. And at times you've got to put your health at the top of the agenda. Because at the end of the day that's going to benefit not just you, but your whole family and everybody around you. But it's a choice that people are too quick to compromise.*
>
> *You've got to be ruthless on the planning. I know that if I stick to the routine, then I'll make time for myself and the things that I also want to do. Exercising is a great example. So, when I map out the week, I instantly think about which days am I going to have time to get into a gym and work out or get outside and do something. For me routine becomes the important factor."*

***

Think of it like this:

It can take a lot of effort to push a clunky car to the top of a hill, but once you've got there and it moves like a new sports car, the effort to maintain speed is minimal:

> *"Your Life does not get better by chance, it gets better by change"*

> – JIM ROHN

USE YOUR HEAD MAN!

HOW MINDFULNESS AND FINDING YOUR COMPASS CAN MAKE YOU A LEGEND

"The definition of insanity is doing the same thing over and over again and expecting different results."

ALBERT EINSTEIN

This is square one. You may be asking yourself what this means and why we aren't looking at the best workout or how only eating baby food will get you shredded? You know, the *real* secrets to becoming a bona fide athlete with a 6-pack.

We will address those things but before we can get into any of the physical we must sort what's going on in your head, for this is the key to it all.

If you remember how insulin was the bouncer to the club of your cells and your pancreas was the club owner, then your brain and mind is the governor, chairman, CEO and President. He knows all. Well, apart from the odd family birthday and house key placement.

A lot of this is on an unconscious level, so for the country to operate effectively the boss must be running at capacity and making all the right calls. Your mind and thoughts determine you as a man, how your body will look and how you'll feel each day.

However, without true desire, drive, and conscious determination to improve and implement the positive changes into your daily life and make them a priority, you'll struggle to get to your end goal. You must have consistent application of the right behaviours and this comes from where your head is at.

For example, you can't lose your gut and still drink booze often.

Can you give up the beers? Do you think you can still drink heavily and shed kilos of fat at the same time? You can't. This is the kind of desire and sacrifice you have to make – booze and the same shit you've always done, *or* getting in awesome shape, feeling fantastic, and *really* enjoying the odd drink.

Remember, no beer tastes as good as being a strong, lean, athletic, and confident Alpha feels.

Along with this desire and commitment to change, we also need to tackle your outlook and approach to daily life. No one is immune to extremes in emotion and bad days, however, what is different is constantly looking at the world through shit-coloured glasses. If the boss runs a country like this would you want to live there? Imagine the overflow into society (that's you).

Focus on your thoughts and you'll come out stronger and better off.

A positive approach can be the difference between you losing that stubborn belly fat or waking up to see it mockingly looking up at you every day. It can certainly mean never finding your inner Alpha and gaining the confidence to speak up to your boss and be resolute to your opinion. It can be the difference between getting the partner of your dreams and being rejected. It *is* the difference between being happy and content and consistently unfulfilled.

Admittedly this might sound a little fluffy, however, let's look at what science has to say. Introducing the revolutionary work of internationally renowned scientist Dr. Masaru Emoto.

In his book *Hidden Messages In Water*, Emoto used high-speed photography to show that crystals formed in frozen water when specific, concentrated thoughts were directed at them. Specifically, water that had been exposed to loving words, music, and thought exhibited brilliant, extravagant and colourful snowflake patterns. This matched similar patterns in water from clear springs.

In stark contrast to this, Emoto also showed that water exposed to negative thoughts, music, and words formed incomplete, asymmetrical patterns with dull colours and matched the patterning of polluted water.

What does this mean for you? Well, considering our bodies are highly complex organisms, containing all sorts of tissue and billions of cells, we're still made up of around 60% water. Emoto showed that these results could affect the water contained inside our bodies and with that play a massive part in our health.

So, if you can influence one of the major components of your body through positive thought then it's best you start using a positive approach to life. Make the decision to change your mind and your body will follow suit.

Start by listing the things you value in life the most, sorting them into priorities and getting some perspective around where you should be spending your energy and time, and what needs to be making its way into your life more.

This will help you gain some invaluable insight into who you are and what drives you. It's also going to help you start looking at life differently, taking a positive approach and learning to value what's good in your life. This is also crucial in forming your desired goals in the next step.

The next thing we must do is **make a choice to change**. So once you have your values and you know what drives you, you need to make a conscious decision to improve yourself. This will be far more manageable when you know a bit more about yourself and attack it with a positive frame of mind.

Start comprehending this: when it comes to what happens in your life, the choice is literally yours. When you let others make your decisions you're living out someone else's plan, not your own. If you want to become a lean beast of an athlete then you must choose that and the actions relevant to get you there- you must find *your own* compass.

Many men make the mistake of not fully committing; "I've been too busy," "My boss is giving me too much work to do," "The Mrs is all over me," etc., and they put the blame on others.

Are you one of those guys? Do you make excuses and shift the blame for your failures to others? Has your choice been to let others determine your fate? Or have you simply made some bad decisions?

Instead of doing this you must make your own choices and use a positive approach, then any failures are yours and yours alone. Own your choices, and own your life.

Your life is a result of the choices you make. If you don't like your life it's time to start making better choices.

The food, training and other key lifestyle choices you make today and every day reflect what your body, health, energy and mind will be in the future. Choose what outcome you want.

When it comes to implementing our positive approach to life and getting started on your journey to looking and feeling great and unleashing your Alpha, I want you to ask yourself a few questions:

- Why are you doing this?
- Who are you doing it for?
- What do you want to gain from it?
- What are your expectations?

- How will you feel ten years from now if nothing changes?
- How will you feel ten years from now if you've ticked this box and moved onto bigger and better things, a life more awesome?

Your mindset is more than just wanting to change. You must have awareness of who you are and what makes you tick. You must become mindful.

***

The next stop for us mastering this part of your journey is for you to think about what it is you actually want. What do you want to achieve? It doesn't have to be one thing, it can be many; and it doesn't have to be for now or next year, it can be 20 years from now. These goals are crucial to you making the commitment and finding the desire to change.

Once you have these, think about who these goals are for. Are these goals really for you, or are they ultimately for someone else? This is key – if they're not for you then you need to readdress and make these goals for yourself and yourself only.

In the end you can only rely on yourself and control *your* actions, true happiness comes from within yourself – so nail this for *you,* and the rest will follow. Find your *own* compass.

The next part of your achievement snowball is setting constant short term goals. These are things you're going to set at the start of every week. These are one of the best ways to inch off bite-size chunks towards your big goals, they also help to keep motivation strong and remind you of what you're doing and why.

Write these down and keep them where you can see them. Tell someone close to you about them, so they can hold you accountable. This little tactic is something that's going to play a huge part in your success. We want to draw from within and for you to be in control of your choices, but having the support and accountability of someone you trust and don't want to disappoint is going to ram home your compliance.

This is delving into the often avoided area of vulnerability, something guys often see as a weakness. However, you are now to replace that thought with one of strength. For, to be vulnerable shows you are strong and secure enough in yourself. This is real inner strength.

This is your next step: choosing someone to keep you accountable and someone you can be open and honest with. Think about this and choose wisely.

It's time now to take those infantile goals and mature them into a vivid picture in your mind. Not everyone's goals will simply be "get to x body fat percentage," which could lend itself to a borrowed picture of someone with that physique.

You might have a goal to have regular sex with your partner again, or you might want a certain position at work that you know is coming up, maybe you want to be in a position where you're confident enough to approach girls without a skin full of beers – and not only chat but get phone numbers.

These can be made all the more powerful if you visualise yourself having attained your goals. Visualisation will help anchor your goals in your mind and get you into a mindset of being there and getting a feeling for what it's like. It will also ensure your behaviours start acting in a way that points you towards them.

Now to really drive this visual home, you're going to write it down, tell a bit of a story of where you have got to, and firmly plant this in your mind. **Make it powerful, descriptive, and inspiring.**

Stick this vision somewhere you'll see it, like next to your bed, so you'll see it often enough for it to start anchoring its way into your thoughts. For this vision to come true you must accept it, want it, and believe it.

One of the aspects of our Alpha is training, eating, and treating yourself like an athlete. Certainly our Alpha looks like an athlete, so if you aim to get in great physical shape – lean, strong, muscular, and confident – then you need to start treating yourself like an athlete.

This simple but powerful quote by *Bill Bowerman,* track and field coach and co-founder of *Nike,* says it all:

"If you have a body, you are an athlete"

***

"The two most important days in your life are the day you were born... and the day you find out why"

– MARK TWAIN

Our next step in using your head is to take your values, your big long-term goals, your vision for your future and use these to flush out what it is you really want from life. What gets you excited? What do you strongly believe in? So strongly that if mentioned you feel you *have* to speak up about it? What pisses you off? Not only this, but it lights a fire inside of you just thinking about it.

Many men have never ever put a single second of thought into this, simply drifting through life from one moment to the next in a "what happens will happen" kind of absent mentality. That's fine if you want to look back on a life of not much at all – a lot of the same with nothing outstanding to account for, having no compass of your own and most likely following someone else's.

However, if you feel like you've got more to give, there's more in this world than just floating along and you'd like to look back on your life with pride and a sense of achievement, then it's time to figure out what it is you really want to do and then **go do it.**

You must find *your own* direction.

Thinking of your "bigger game" can have a powerful effect. When you think, **"I'm doing big things"** it changes you and how you look at things. You start to think of what's possible in situations, which is a powerful thing, especially when inserted into your own life and goals, but when it becomes bigger than you it holds huge power.

A mission is what you do every minute of every day (or at least where those things are taking you). It lights you up and gives your life and every day, purpose and possibility.

Here's a great perspective on this from the late Steve Jobs:

"For the past 33 years, I have looked in the mirror every morning and asked myself: 'If today were the last day of my life, would I want to do what I am about to do today?' And whenever the answer has been 'No' for too many days in a row, I know I need to change something."

Once you have this you need to work on it, refine it and keep ensuring it fits your top values and that it excites you. This powerful thought process won't just have a massive effect on your mindset, it's going to pave the way for you to unleash your inner Alpha – what we're here for!

Then whatever your goals may be, you have the foundation set and the blueprint to build the rest.

Even the ancient thinkers had this stuff nailed. Aristotle

pinpointed with this quote way back...

"We are what we repeatedly do. Excellence then, is not act, but a habit."

Not only is finding your passion going to bring new and long term happiness to your life due to the fact that you'll be spending large amounts of time doing something you love, it's also used by leading experts, such as Dr Phillips, to positively affect one's mental health:

"One of the major tap roots we have as men is our work, our profession, what we do. And one should always try to find something special in what one does. It doesn't matter whether you're the prime minister or clean a gutter. The important thing is to find meaning in what you do. And if you can, that is worth an awful lot in terms of one's mental health."

Here's Steve Jobs again with some awesome insight and the kind of approach that can help us men:

"Your work is going to fill a large part of your life, and the only way to be truly satisfied is to do what you believe is great work. And the only way to do great work is to love what you do. If you haven't found it yet, keep looking, and don't settle. As with all matters of the heart... you'll know when you find it"

Follow your destiny, not someone else's and ensure your goals fit *you*. Ponder this quote from nutritional and obesity expert Dr. Yoni Freedhoff:

"Your real goal? Live the healthiest life you can enjoy, not the healthiest life you can tolerate. Yes, if you have weight to lose, you'll have to make changes. But if you change so far from who you are and what you enjoy, odds are that it's not a sustainable plan. Don't aim for your so-called 'ideal' weight; instead aim for what I refer to as your 'best' weight, which is the weight you reach when living the healthiest life you can actually enjoy."

Set goals and make them specific. If you have body composition goals then you must measure where you are now. If you have access I recommend getting a thorough body composition DEXA scan. This will provide you with a clear picture of where you are now and new scans will let you know your progress. Outside of this take pictures and measurements.

Take home point: You must have patience when it comes to your long-term goals. If for example you're currently carrying an extra 15 kilograms of body fat. Then you need to lose this and it's going to take some time.

However, if you set your mind to it and make the right habitual lifestyle changes *you will get there*.

Patience can be tough to come by but you must have it in spades and match it with your determination, hard work, positivity, dedication, application and consistency.

Think of it like this: if you're carrying that extra 15 kilos and you're 40 years-old, then it's safe enough to assume that you probably put that weight on over about 15-20 years. **That's a long time!** Your mission and journey to lose that spare tyre and ultimately unleash your inner Alpha will take a *fraction* of that 15-20 years.

You can make giant strides to living the life *you* want in no time. Certainly in one year from now you can look back thanking yourself for deciding to change and doing the hard work to get to the awesomeness you're now at.

And that's great news, right?

All it requires is *application*. Sure, the choice and control that we spoke about earlier has to be there, but applying it is the follow through. What good is a game plan without it being played out?

It's time to follow through on your plans.

"What would life be like if we had no courage to attempt anything?"

– VINCENT VAN GOGH

MINDSET TASKS

Task one: Your core values and what you're grateful for

Start a gratitude journal. Do this today and every day for one week to start. Do this before bed or upon waking in the morning. This is so you start taking specific note of the awesome things in your life to ensure your mindset and outlook is positive where possible. No matter how big or small, be grateful. Even try to practise it in times of frustration and anger.

Next come your core values. Start listing the values that you treasure. What words come to mind when you see the good in people and yourself? When someone pisses you off, what characteristic have they not showed that you think is important? List as many as possible, then come back to it and define your top 5 values, the things that you give the most weight in life.

Task two: Goal setting

All goals, both short and long term must be a combination

of outcome and behavioural. For example, an outcome goal would be drop 5 kg of body fat; so complementary behavioural goals would be things like training 5 times per week, preparing my meals each day with vegetables and meats in each meal and getting 7 hours quality sleep per night. Those constant behaviours, when achieved, will help you achieve the outcome goal of dropping fat. Outcomes must have behaviours attached.

You're going to set some S.M.A.R.T. goals, which means they must be:

- **S**pecific
- **M**easurable
- **A**chievable
- **R**ealistic
- **T**imed

Now take the terms *achievable* and *realistic* and stretch them out to be slightly *over the top*. So you're really setting **SMOT** goals. They'll be achievable and realistic, but you're going to aim high and make it something you really have to strive for.

Put down as many as you like and you can come back and refine them until you have something that rings true with you and lights you up. These goals need to set your spirit alight so you have no choice but to choose the right course of action *and* apply yourself in the way needed to achieve them. Get carried away if need be, but make sure they fall into the categories above.

Do this for the next 12-16 weeks and also 9-12 months.

Now, *make a promise to yourself that you will achieve these goals.* Get a piece of paper and write down your goals and make a contract. Think of something that you'd love to get yourself if you achieve the biggest goal. Scale it down and do it for all the smaller ones too.

Now agree on a consequence if you don't achieve them, *but make it positive and worthwhile.* For example if you don't achieve 'X' you will donate $100 to 'Y' charity, and so on. Sign it and have someone witness and sign it too.

Task three: Short term goals and little wins

Each week you're going to set two goals that can be measured and achieved. For example, "This week I will train 5 times for more than 30 minutes. I will also have 6 alcohol free days this week with a maximum of 5 standard drinks total." As with your big goals, put something on it – for example, if one is missed have a contract with yourself that you'll do another interval session, or have zero drinks next week. For the most part make these behavioural and specific– e.g., drinking 2 litres of water/day – as opposed to "staying hydrated."

Make sure you recognise and celebrate these little wins. That doesn't mean splurge and reward yourself with crap food – you're not a Labrador – but ensure you get in a habit of identifying these wins; they help build and maintain your positive energy while chipping away at the big guys. Write these little wins down each week.

Task four: Accountability and honesty

Choose someone that you trust and confide in, that's willing to be a big part of your journey, but also be tough on you. This person is going to be your external accountability. Even better if this person is making a similar change in their life.

Tell them your goals, both large and small. You're going to check in with them *each week* (even daily) and share what you're working on that week, how you've been, how you've gone with your weekly goals, and how you're progressing with your long-term goals. You need to be honest with them and share any troubles or roadblocks you may come to, however, make sure you also share all the positives and little wins you have.

Choose your person carefully. "One of the boys" might not be a good choice, depending on what your mates are like. If they're anything like most, you might get more shit than encouragement, so choose wisely. Your partner/wife/significant other also might not work the best, as they can be supportive and dangerous at the same time.

Outline what you're doing and that you wish to debrief with them for 10-20 minutes every week. In person if possible, but over the phone or Skype will work. They need to be fully on board – daily text messages work well.

Task five: Visualisation and 5-year anchor

Start with the date 5 years from now and detail where you'll be, what your day is like, how it makes you feel, and how you feel about life in general. Get some clear visuals of what you'll look like, how you'll feel and where you'll be once you reach them. This should excite you. Then write this vision down. Outline what makes you happy. Now, write this out in pen every day for a week. After that read once a day every day.

Next, take this end goal – this vision of your life – and *list 100 ways in which achieving this will serve your top 5 values* from earlier. Keep going until you hit a blank, then push through two more blanks and see what you can get down. We want you to nail home why achieving this goal is the only option for you and hone in on your drive to get there.

Try splitting into these categories if it will make it easier: mental/learning, career, financial, family, social, physical, and spiritual.

Task six: Your mission and driving passion

Think about your values and your ultimate goals. Now think about the rest of your life and what you do – does it make you happy? What does? *Now look ahead with this and ask what do I want to be known for?* If you can unlock what it is that really excites and drives you, even what pisses you off and how you want to be remembered, then you'll start unravelling your passion and what your mission in life is. It might mean some tough life decisions - so be it - plan and execute. This is vitally important stuff remember- *it's your life!*

> *"People do not decide to become extraordinary. They decide to accomplish extraordinary things."*
>
> – SIR EDMUND HILLARY

Get to work on these, keep notes, come back to it from time to time, refine, adjust, and shift whatever needs it. Get clear on what you want your life to be and **go do it.**

> *"Whatever you want to do, do it. There are only so many tomorrows"*
>
> – MICHAEL LANDON

HOW TO EAT LIKE A MAN
FOOD, DRINK AND NUTRITION FOR TODAY'S ALPHA

"Dis-moi ce que tu manges, je te dirai ce que tu es."
(Tell me what you eat and I will tell you what you are)

– ANTHELME BRILLAT-SAVARIN, 1826

Food is the area that lets most men down, or, more accurately, most men *let themselves down* with food. As we've seen in the previous chapter we must start by approaching things in the right way mentally, but nutrition is either your biggest tool or your worst enemy.

Done wrong and this can be a waistline, health, and libido killer. Done right and it can be a fat burning, muscle building, Alpha making weapon.

Taking the easy way out is all too common, however, it doesn't have to be that way. This is your simple guide to attacking nutrition the way a man should. This will not only help you create and maintain a lean, strong and muscular body, but it will help you to sleep better, have more energy and concentration, increase libido, and set you up to be a healthy man – a true Alpha.

As the long gone Frenchman above said: *you are what you eat*.

So we've spoken about where your head's at and how

mindfulness will initiate and strengthen your journey. If you want to look like an athlete then you need to start treating yourself like one. This goes for nutrition too. To look like an athlete you must start eating as if you are one, ergo, if you eat like an athlete you become one. Eat like a gluttonous slob and hey ho, you'll be one!

This is most pertinent when it comes to health. Food is often thought as a tasty necessity to be eaten at intervals throughout the day and nothing more. Often included in social settings such as "catch ups" and meetings, it becomes a huge struggle for people to manage these social situations and their eating. The social pressure to conform and eat normally is huge. This resultantly throws people off the wagon or never allows them on it to begin with.

This is something you must shake now. Excuses for others opinions and beliefs are just that, excuses. Make your **own** choices and be responsible for your actions.

To Unleash Your Alpha you must eat only the best where possible and the best you will become.

In today's society food is not given the credit it's due. What food and drink goes in your mouth is largely what your body becomes. There are other factors obviously and luckily for you we're covering them inside these pages. However, food plays such a vital role in not only fuelling your body with energy for movement, but in providing all the elements your body needs for its day-to-day functioning.

If your nutrition is poor, no matter the training you do, you won't achieve your body, health, or performance potential. The same is true for your health.

Changes in your body whether it be increasing muscle, decreasing fat, or attaining great health will not happen unless you're giving your body the correct nutrients and building blocks for change.

Food is your number one stop for healthcare.

Eat to fuel your body and it will respond with great health and a six-pack.

Too often food is an afterthought and doesn't appear on people's radars as a key element for health and disease prevention. Think back to all those conditions and chronic diseases we spoke about earlier which are in horrific abundance such as obesity, diabetes, depression and heart disease; getting your nutrition right can not only prevent these but help rid your body of them!

Modern day health care could more accurately be called *"sick care,"* targeted at *treating* illness and disease **more so than preventing it.** Sadly, it's often a case of "the horse has already bolted," whereas a healthy approach to nutrition will put you in the best stead for living an awesome, healthy life and avoiding illness and chronic disease. Oh yeah, and looking lean and ripped!

The good news is, *it's not that hard!*

My simple nutritional philosophies are:
Eat real, nutrient dense food. If it was growing or moving around as naturally as possible then it's mostly fair game. This means:

- Quality meat from animals that lived a cruisy life in their natural environment; beef from cattle that walked around grassy paddocks, chicken from birds that cruised the pastures, etc.
- Plenty of quality vegetables especially greens. Fruit daily, especially berries. Ensure to wash all produce
- A small amount of raw nuts each day
- Fresh and free range eggs from the chilled out kind of birds mentioned above

- A variety of quality fats; from animals in small amounts, avocado, extra virgin olive oil on salads, pasture fed butter on greens, coconut oil to cook with, omega 3s from fish (and supplemental)
- Dairy as natural as possible – this means raw full fat milk (or unhomogenised), organic and natural/Greek yoghurt – no added sugar
- Drink plenty of water consistently throughout the day
- Drink plenty of green and white tea and one to two black coffees per day – nothing after 2pm

Avoid: unnatural and processed foods, large amounts of alcohol, sugar and refined carbohydrates such as flour and wheat as much as possible:

- Food in packets should be minimized and always check the ingredients list for unwanted nasties
- Use supplements to fill holes where needed and appropriate
- Plan, prepare, and prosper
- Every now and then relax and do whatever you want

These are summed up very nicely for me with this awesome little quote from Ann Wigmore, one of the earliest modern pioneers on nutrition and healthy living:

"The food you eat can be either the safest and most powerful form of medicine or the slowest form of poison"

- ANN WIGMORE

This is supposed to be simple right? We aren't going to get complicated and dive into amounts and percentages of total daily energy intake, calories, etc. We must first get the food choices right. The amounts will sort themselves out once we implement a few key strategies later on.

You should never have to count a calorie.

***

Should I eat organic?

Organic is a tricky one. It could be essential, depending on where you live, or not a concern at all. At the very least start learning how and what to look for and who to ask.

When buying meat ask your butcher if the beef is grass-fed. If it's not, or they can't or won't tell you, find a new butcher. Same for fishmongers – is it fresh? Is that salmon farmed (in which case avoid)?

You'll often end up paying more for better quality, but as 11 year-old Birke Baehr put it when he gave an inspirational talk on sustainable and natural farming, "*You pay the farmer, or you pay the hospital.*" So pay more cash now or pay big time later on with your health and body composition.

Nutrition for optimal health, body composition, athletic performance and general daily functioning of our Alpha **must include quality proteins, quality carbs, and quality fats.** So before you go wasting thought on perplexing good fat choices and macronutrient levels we need to consider the quality of all our food sources. This is how you get in **real shape and unleash your athletic Alpha.**

The ultimate nutrition to get you lean, defined, strong and healthy contains **quality** protein sources, **quality** carbohydrate sources, and **quality** fat sources. This has to be the starting point for all nutrition plans.

This is much more than our calorie in/calorie out simplicity. This is where your hormones come in again. We want to

maximise these with nutrition too.

Before we get into your nutritional table of good and bad choices, make sure you're filling out your food diary. Keeping a real honest track is the only way forward.

We'll get into some specific fat loss and muscle building plans later, but first let's take a look at what's good and what's not so good. Below I have outlined a quick and easy table to get you going:

PROTEIN		FAT		CARBOHYDRATE	
GOOD	NOT SO GOOD	GOOD	NOT SO GOOD	GOOD	NOT SO GOOD
Farmed meat pasture/grass fed/raised (walked around)	Grain fed & hormone/ antibiotic treated & mass produced meat – 'factory farmed'	Animal fat from healthy animals in small amounts	Vegetable oils e.g. Canola, sunflower	Leafy green and coloured vegetables	Sugar & refined grains e.g. flour
Wild game	Processed meat e.g. hotdogs, commercial deli meats, pies	Coconut oil-extra virgin cold pressed (cooking)	Cooking with olive oil	Root veggies e.g. Sweet potato, pumpkin, carrot, beets	White potato often
Wild fish	Farmed salmon	Grass fed Butter/ghee	Margarines	Quinoa	Bread, buns
Free range organic eggs	Cage eggs	Avocado	Processed low fat foods	Buckwheat	Pasta
Raw/natural dairy (organic full fat un-homogenised)	Low fat/ heavily processed dairy	Fish oil from wild fish/wild krill oil	Cheap fish oils	Black, brown or wild rice	Noodles, white rice
Pure cold filtered protein powders- WPI, WPC, casein	Protein supplements containing ingredients you can't pronounce...	Olive oil- extra virgin (to dress), macadamia oil, avocado oil	Highly processed seed oils including trans fats	Fruit especially berries and dark skin fruits	Biscuits, crackers, rice cakes, muffins etc
Legumes, nuts in small amounts	Soy products such as tofu	Raw nuts/raw nut butters	Peanut butter (most)	Fresh dates, naturally dried fruit (no preservatives)	Cereals, muesli
		Free range organic eggs	Cage eggs, not eating yolk		

Note: **ingredients on food labels are listed with the highest content ingredient first and then so on.**

We'll delve more into amounts and serving sizes later in more detail, but for now you need to focus on learning how much you need to eat by *listening to your body*.

What this means is when we blindly get stuck into a meal and pay no attention to either how much we're eating or the speed at which we're eating it, we invariably eat too much. Not only that, but our digestive systems can't handle being fed quickly with partly chewed food.

Think for a second, do you ever get gas? This is often due to food intolerances and their reactions in your gut, but also too much food that hasn't been chewed properly. Eating quickly and not chewing fully result in too much food being eaten and your gut struggling to handle what it's receiving. Various adverse effects can result, such as bloating in the acute stages and fat storage in the latter stages. Not good for our Alpha.

Your hormonal and nervous systems determine what functions your body is going to prioritise at any given time. If your parasympathetic nervous system (PNS) is on you'll be in "rest and digest" mode, if you're "on the go," mentally or physically, your sympathetic nervous system (SNS) or 'fight or flight' is on and you won't be digesting properly.

One very important thing to note is that most of your immune system receptor cells are found in your digestive system, so when this is compromised such as the example above, fat storage is the least of your worries. Slowly your body's defence against disease and petty illness like cold and flu is beaten into submission. Poor body composition is the end result.

For your body to digest and absorb the nutrients from the food you eat *you must take your time, eat slowly, and relax. Try not to get distracted, but actually focus on eating.*

Think of it like this:

- If your goal is to shed fat then think about this delicious food doing just that
- If your goal is to increase lean muscle think about this lovely animal helping do exactly that
- If your goal is to increase energy and overall health then simply put some thought into the food you're eating and the wonderful nutrition you're getting from it

And so on. It may sound a little bit "let's hold hands and chant" but believe me, when you're eating, this is the best state to be in to burn fat, build lean muscle, and simply move closer to being more awesome.

"EVERYONE has a six pack; you just have to expose it" <=== Tweet that! @mcampbell2012 #UnleashYourAlpha

***

Let's take a look at our main three nutrients, our macronutrients.

FAT

First, what about these mysterious "good fats?"

We're afraid of fat. We hold it at arm's length thinking, "It's got **fat** in it, which means it'll be in me and *I'll get fat*!" Well, when it comes to eating fat, quality fat choices is the key.

Some fats are amazing for us. They provide us with energy, nutrients, and all sorts of supportive additions to our bodies proper functioning. On the other hand, some are rubbish and may as well be labelled poison.

Keep fats simple:

Haves
- Extra virgin coconut oil for cooking and smoothies, etc.
- Extra virgin olive oil for dressings and marinades (do not use to cook on medium-high heats)
- Animal fat on meat, eggs, etc. Chicken skin, steak, duck fat for cooking
- Butter from pasture fed cows to dress veggies (cooking only on low heats), ghee (cooking)
- Raw nuts
- Avocado
- Fish oil for supplementation

Avoids
- Vegetable oils, such as canola oil, sunflower oil, soybean oil, cottonseed oil
- Trans fats
- Margarines and non-butter spreads
- Eggs from caged hens
- Processed packaged foods that largely contain vegetable oils to some degree

Outside of this seek out the advice of an expert.

Saturated fat in particular is painted as the bad guy that will not only make you a fatty, but *kill you*. Like Elvis and his infamous "hollowed out loaf of bread stuffed with bacon and peanut butter then deep fried," most things in excess aren't great for you. However, in the right amounts saturated fat is downright awesome for you.

I've had countless clients leave the fat on their steak, put butter on greens, olive oil on salads, and cook with coconut oil in and continue to lose fat, put on muscle, and function at their best. That's why we're here, right?

PROTEIN

What are healthy, quality protein choices?

The opinion of many very respected people in the health and nutrition field is that meat (beef, lamb, poultry, and seafood) is the best bang for your buck protein source. Not only this, but it has many other amazing *and* crucial nutrients we need as humans.

Animals raised in the most natural way possible are vital. If it walked around, swam, or flew as nature intended, have at it. If it was cooped up or fed something different to what it would eat in the wild, *seriously avoid*. It's as bad as processed meat and grains. Ask your suppliers if you're not sure.

This goes for things like grain fed beef, farmed fish and cage chicken/eggs.

Same goes for soy products like tofu. If it's highly messed around with, full of preservatives, horrible trans fats, sugars, and words that seem better suited to a pharmacy or a Chernobyl documentary then **avoid!**

There's plenty of amazing bacon, ham, and sausages out there, but you need to source quality options that are free from harmful additives. Find a good butcher who sells quality products and ask them the right questions, such as, "Is this bacon preservative/nitrate free?"

Your body isn't designed to break down copious foreign chemicals and manufactured things like preservatives and vegetable oils. These take up vital energy and resources when introduced into the body and can cause massive cellular damage through a number of complex reactions that your body simply a) can do without, and b) sees as unfamiliar as a vegan in a slaughterhouse. They're bad for your body, plain and simple.

Dairy products should be in small amounts and as natural as possible. That means raw milk and cheese, unpasteurized and unhomogenised if possible. However, organic full fat and unhomogenised milk is second choice, *but in small amounts*. If you seem to handle it well, then you can probably afford to have a bit more.

When it comes to yoghurt go for organic/biodynamic pot set yoghurt or Greek yoghurt without added sugar. Commercial milk and dairy products that have been messed around with by harsh processing techniques are lacking in nutrients. They also lack quality enzymes that help process lactose, hence why so many people have a problem when they drink 'normal' milk. Plus, natural milk just tastes better!

Protein powder supplements: see your supplementation bonus material.

CARBOHYDRATES

What are healthy, quality carbohydrate options then?

This is tricky. There are many arguments concerning this subject, from archaic, simple-minded opinions to drastic cut all-measures views to science-laden monotonous perspectives.

'Carbs are good, eat more wholegrains'. 'Sugar is evil and should be avoided at all costs'. 'Bread will make you fat'. 'Eat only slow releasing carbs to help you feel fuller for longer'.

It's time to stop listening to the noise.

There are indeed some very poor carbohydrate options, just like there are some amazingly beneficial and crucial ones. The key is first having the simple ground rules and then applying the relevant dimensions to **you.** Fine-tuning is for another time.

Here are your quality carbohydrate sources:

Greens and vegetables are number one. Not only packed full of nutrients, but greens in particular will help you alkalize the body and fight inflammation and cellular damage. These along with coloured vegetables provide quality carbohydrates and copious vitamins and minerals. Starchy vegetables, for the most part whilst dropping body fat, are for training days. Simple.

***

Do not stick with what you've always done and simply wait and hope for things to change – create change! **Ensure all of your food options are quality! Good fats, good proteins, and good carbs.** Give your body its best chance.

This is a wonderful place to execute some of those short-term goals from earlier. You may find it difficult to completely overhaul your eating from what it currently is to my recommendations, so set small weekly behavioural goals to make one or two changes at a time. For example:

- This week I will eat naturally raised meat
- This week I will eat greens with every meal
- This week I will eat 5 cups of veggies a day

Putting in the effort now and making it consistent will ultimately be immensely rewarding and make maintaining your athletic Alpha body much easier than getting to that point, but you must apply yourself and have patience.

***

We don't just eat nutrition, we drink it too. The term "empty calories" is sometimes used with some beverages. However, that implies that it's purely not beneficial. It doesn't indicate that it's actually detrimental. Perhaps the term *"harmful calories"* would be better.

Soft drinks, alcohol, sports drinks, and anything that isn't essentially natural is a great way to screw up your solid food nutritional work. Eliminate. Life balance and a little booze can most definitely re-enter in time but to create this initial change it must be seriously limited for now. The rest can stay out.

Hydration is crucial for your cells to function optimally. Without it, the country (that's you remember) is in drought.

My recommendations for fluid intake are:

Water: Drink plenty of water throughout the day. Make sure this is consistent and not just drinking a lot at once – it must be sipped on regularly. Also, I recommend slightly salting your drinking water; *you shouldn't be able to taste the salt.* In short, this ensures that the water we drink is taken into the cells in our bodies so we can use it better and contains beneficial minerals. Use only quality rock salt or sea salt, *not* table salt (This goes for salting anything).

Coffee: Limit to a maximum of 2 per day and *nothing past 2 pm or after training.* If possible ensure the beans are organic, as most non-organic beans are *heavily* sprayed with toxins. Limit the milk in your coffee as much as possible – try switching to long blacks, macchiatos, and espressos. Even try a long black with a *dash* of heavy cream or coconut oil, and cinnamon – this is gold! Before training coffee is a great stimulant and mobilises free fatty acids to be used as fuel. After training it will act to promote a catabolic state – *so try and avoid!*

Tea: Green tea and white tea are full of beneficial antioxidants. *I recommend drinking at least 2 cups per day* to help fight cellular damage and help burn fat. Note: White tea is a type of tea, not black tea with milk. I also use this cold as the liquid addition to smoothies.

Milk: If possible have raw dairy. That means _un_pasteurised and _un_homogenised. If you can get it then include in your week, if not you can use organic unhomogenised in small amounts. Avoid almond/rice/soy milks as they usually contain a lot of unwanted crap, or make your own almond milk.

Coconut water: This is the natural juice of a young coconut and is an amazing natural hydrator. I recommend using this on days of heavy exercise as a way to re-hydrate. Stay away from "sports drinks" as much as possible, but use this in moderation. Try adding to your post workout shake instead of water.

Apple cider vinegar (with 'The Mother'): This harks back to the work on your gut health. Apple cider vinegar is an awesome addition to salad dressing, a cup of tea, or water. It's a harsh taste for some but a great way to stimulate your gut and aid digestion.

Bone broths and stocks: This means homemade, however, not necessarily by you. Many butchers and small deli style stores sell homemade versions. These guys contain all the amazing nutrition from the bones of the animal and are a tremendous addition to any diet, be it shredding, gaining muscle or just seeking great health.

AVOID: Most other drinks! Depending on your goals and current body composition. However, I strongly recommend that *the next 16 weeks be an alcohol free zone!* If in doubt leave it out.

***

As a very wise man Hippocrates once said, **"Let your food be thy medicine, and your medicine be thy food."** From there you can be whatever man you want to be.

Time to make some sacrifices, start the hard work and implement the nutritional key points so this can BECOME a lot easier and simply part of your everyday life.

It's time to start pushing the car to speed...

NUTRITIONAL KEY POINTS

Key point 1: Be educated as to the right choices and make them with *quality* food. If you're not sure of its origin ask the supplier, otherwise go organic. Remove all bad options from your fridge and cupboard. Stock only quality options.

Key point 2: Eat slowly until *satisfied, not stuffed.* Putting your knife and fork down between mouthfuls and chewing properly are absolute keys to discovering how much to eat. This not only helps you with how much to eat, but is the first and most important step in digesting and absorbing the nutrients from your food**.**

Key point 3: Fat sources – Coconut oil, avocado, olive oil, butter, nuts, eggs, animal fats. Products like margarines that "lower your cholesterol" and claim to be good for your heart are not! Nor are "low fat" or "no fat" options. If the fat (that was most likely beneficial to begin with) has been removed then this food no doubt contains chemicals and sugar that will actually cause damage!

Other fats are hugely beneficial and must be included in your diet – don't be afraid of fats, just ensure you're having the right ones in moderation.

Key point 4: How an animal lived its life not only affects the taste, but it is vitally important to the quality of the meat it produces. This has the direct effect on your physical and mental health and body composition.

Key point 5: Protein sources – Meat from naturally raised, pasture-fed, or wild animals and fish. Free-range organic eggs from free range pasture raised chickens, raw nuts, raw natural organic dairy products, and pure protein powders.

Key point 6: Processed sugars and refined carbs such as flour are to be avoided as much as possible. These will not only mess with your body composition and see you gaining body fat but will have you heading further down the road towards the anti-Alpha. The best thing you can do for your health and body now and long term is largely remove these from your diet.

Key point 7: Carb sources – Leafy greens in large amounts and coloured vegetables with every meal, fruits daily, root vegetables especially sweet potato, buckwheat, and quinoa on training days (post workout in particular).

Key point 8: If it's processed, contains preservatives and has been altered from its natural state to get to your mouth, leave it out where possible! Choose quality food options.

Key point 9: Fluids – Water, black coffee, teas, raw/unprocessed natural milk, coconut water, apple cider vinegar. Avoid most other drinks, including booze in large amounts.

The following steps are from the bonus material in the appendix of this book. This is your specific fat burning and muscle building information.

Key point 10: Your number 1 food preparation strategy is cooking in bulk. This will work differently if you're cooking for yourself or others also, but the main thing to do is add 2 servings to what you need to cook and these bad boys will serve you tomorrow. *Cook extra at night for the next day. Have your meals ready to go in easily manageable containers.* It's that easy.

Key point 11: Pay attention to when your body is hungry and in need of food. If not then don't force yourself to eat. This should be 2-5 meals per day, with the same amount of food being spread among them regardless. Post training you must have some protein with a small amount of fruit inside the first hour. Otherwise, ensure protein and veggies with every meal, starchy carbs on training days post workout and fats in small amounts in other meals.

Key point 12: Meal serving sizes will vary depending on meal timing. If you eat 3 times per day they will be slightly bigger than if you eat 4 times and bigger again if you eat 5 times.

Think of your plate as a pie chart. *Protein will be about 25%, vegetables will be about 60-65% and fat will be 10-15% (Berardi, 2011). See below:*

NORMAL MEAL SERVING PROPORTIONS

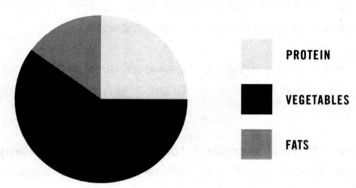

As opposed to post workout that will be bigger in size and have proportions that look more like this:

POST WORKOUT MEAL PROPORTIONS

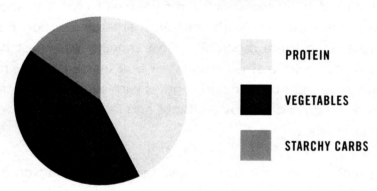

Note that starchy carbs have replaced fats here.

Key point 13: Always have options near work and home that you can use if your normal eating can't happen as per the plan. There will be times when it's hard to avoid, but the more you can control your meals the better progress you'll make towards seeing your six pack.

Find 5 'go-to' places near home and work. Also reach for the kettle and tea bags as a hunger breaker. The main aim here is to differentiate between actual hunger and a want to eat – **two very different things.**

Key point 14: Once a week have a relaxed meal to allow yourself a little break. However, ensure it's only one and still contains most of our key elements to help reinforce your new habits. Adding more relaxed meals will definitely come after your initial 12-16 weeks with more balance and less need for wholesale change in your body and hormones.

Key point 15: Fall off the wagon gently – don't let one slip up derail your entire day or week. Get straight back into your good habits and count this as your relaxed meal for the week. If this was scheduled elsewhere, simply substitute it. If you've already had it that week, remove next week's. *Make sure you enjoy the pants off it though!*

Key point 16: If you're going somewhere that you know serves crap food or this is a possibility (even at a mate's house), have a salad before you go. To quote celebrity chef and nutritionist Pete Evans: *"Fill up on good stuff so there's no room for bad."* Simple.

Key point 17: Balance in life and nutrition is important, so lay the foundations with the above but make sure to relax and let yourself eat whatever you'd like every now and then. Just control it to a rarity, especially when dropping body fat.

Now that you've read the basic information, it's time to get you instigating your nutrition plan.

FOLLOW THESE STEPS OVER THE NEXT 16 WEEKS:

1. Food diary: Complete your food diary for 2 weeks. Pay close attention to the content, amounts, and specific meal macronutrient breakdown. We want you to get an idea through the information above and your diary as to what you need to add or take out.

2. Meal plan: Next is to design a food plan for one week, after the 2 weeks of journaling. I have provided one in the appendix, but the idea is that you become able to make these choices yourself using the simple information and nutritional take home points provided.

So give it a crack and then once you've done it, *and only once you've done it*, have a look at the sample and see how they compare. Certainly the actual contents will differ, however, the key is the type of food and nutrient sources that you use e.g., protein, fat, vegetables, etc.

3. Mental meal plan: Once you've planned a week and followed through on it, then altered where needed and done one more week's worth, we want to try and slowly wean you off the diary. So now you're going to take the written plan and try to do this in your head when you go shopping and cook in bulk at the start of the week. From this point on, we want to run a "mental meal plan," with you keeping a check on things mentally, without having to bother with writing things down. Develop this skill and you'll be much better off long-term.

4. Food diary check in: Make this a couple of days every now and then as a check in. The aim is that you have a much better grasp of what to eat, how much, and when. You mentally plan your eating for the week including more relaxed meals and then every now and then you keep your diary to help pinpoint if there's anything sneaking back in too much, or what you may be missing etc.

As mentioned, if you're better suited to 3 meals then spread the food over 3 meals, and so on. Your training may be in the place of one of these small meals.

TIME	MONDAY	TUESDAY	WEDNESDAY	THURSDAY	FRIDAY	SATURDAY	SUNDAY
Breakfast: 6:30am							
2nd Breaky: 10am							
Lunch: 2pm							
2nd Lunch: 4pm							
Dinner: 7:30pm							
Post workout							

There are some dietary techniques and eating styles that involve different content and meal timings that can be very successful. However, they're beyond the scope of this book.

Once you've established some quality and lasting habits following this program then you can try moving into things like *Intermittent Fasting*. For now, in congruence with the other elements of this book, this approach will get you dropping body fat, increasing lean muscle mass and it will transition your inner athletic Alpha to one who eats real, natural whole foods regularly whilst also enjoying each meal.

Always remember that regardless of your short term or long term goals, health must be on your list of priorities, for a healthy man can make his body what he wishes. With health comes flexibility and options – you can shred from 12% body fat to 9% and look like an athlete when you step onto the beach. You can get lean and strong with defined muscle bulk. You can have great energy, no slumps mid-morning and afternoon, have a strong and healthy sex drive, great inner confidence, and a body and life that you love. You can be more awesome.

TRAIN LIKE A BEAST

CHISELLING A MAN INSIDE AND OUT

"Strength does not come from physical capacity. It comes from an indomitable will."

-MAHATMA GANDHI

Let me start by saying you'll no longer be exercising. Exercising is for the elderly and ridiculous infomercials that only ever contain jacked and ripped units who've never used the apparatus in the ad to "exercise."

From now on you'll be ***training.*** Training isn't just exercising – it's an overall philosophy and approach to movement. It implies that you're doing more than moving for the sake of it, but you're **working towards something.**

Regardless of your goals, by now you all have them. Training is a big part of getting there. We start these in the kitchen, as we saw with *How To Eat Like A Man,* and we sculpt and fine-tune them when we train.

That doesn't mean we only hit the gym. There are many different approaches to training – sometimes goal specifics will determine the best course of action.

We're going to keep things nice and simple because even though there are endless options on how best to train and every trainer under the sun has their own best practice; many of these will contradict each other.

When it boils down to it, each man's specific goals and needs determine not only what exercises to do, but in what format and training style. However, for the most part that's irrelevant because men simply need to *move*. Move often, with purpose and intensity.

EVERYONE needs to have a good level of strength and cardiovascular fitness.

We'll go through some simple yet effective and tough programs to get you first on track, then to your destination. After that, specific goals can be more accurately addressed and achieved. Something we focus on in my online coaching program in depth.

We've seen the downsides of the current state of men – shitty hormones, chronic disease, obesity, infertility, low sex drive, ego, lack of direction, unhappiness, fear of failure, depression – these are the exact reasons we need to train and train effectively.

Turning these around are by-products of increasing your fitness, drastically improving your hormonal profile, dropping extra body fat, increasing muscle mass, and maintaining adequate flexibility and mobility.

No one usually wants to think about getting old, but the more work you do now, the better you'll be to rock out as an older Alpha, as well as being in awesome shape now.

Maintaining a low and ideal body fat percentage (let's say 10-12%) will not only allow your hormones to function normally but the cycle flows back: good hormones = good body. The same goes for maintaining a good level of lean muscle mass, healthy bone mineral density and connective tissue. A lean, strong and muscular body will put you in the best position to take charge of your life. You will live large, kick goals on a daily basis, and be a man with confidence, energy, and his shit sorted.

Keeping training simple is all well and good, we know that when in conjunction with optimal nutrition and other lifestyle factors, results come. However, what's really happening in your body is far from simple.

The internal systems, reactions, and workings of your body are incredibly complex. Think of the Universe and its complexity and then put that inside your body. Now you're getting close.

Here's a little science, put simply:

This is where you need to remember back to our hormones from earlier. To promote any beneficial training or body composition change, hormones *must* be addressed and considered.

We want to promote a hormonal environment conducive to results. The right training will work to get all these processes happening inside your body. This is going to be a combination of hypertrophy and strength training, high intensity interval training, metabolic resistance training, and adequate recovery.

Turn to the back of this section for your training key points and programs. I've also gone into more details on these in your downloadable Bonus Training Start Up Guide.

These training styles have been chosen because of the amazing and varied benefits they bring when performed properly:

- Burn unwanted body fat,
- Increase lean muscle, strength, and power
- Increased fitness and endurance
- Increased mobility and stability
- Increased energy, sex drive, and vitality.

You'll see better mood and concentration as well as improved mental health and endless improvements to your overall health and wellbeing.

***

Strength, for example, is such an under rated element in today's men that we're largely a group of weak and unhealthy anti-Alphas.

Those who respect and admire the human form can recognise that large and obese is unhealthy, if nothing else. While skinny, shapeless and floppy is unattractive and unhealthy.

So gents, if you're a gym goer or exercise regularly and you're not lifting, then locate your balls – it's time to begin!

This is also a shout-out to those "weekend warriors" that hit the weights hard but don't seem to change shape or strength and have nagging injuries. Doing the same old routine week in and week out is ineffective at best.

Stagnation is common in the weights room – if you're not progressing, change something<=== Tweet that shit! @mcampbell2012 #UnleashYourAlpha

Proper resistance training is one thing you'll become very familiar with, the next is working your arse off. We don't want to spend hours upon hours in the gym – we want you to be time efficient training beasts.

The foundation of a healthy man lies in internal happiness and drive, low stress, good sleeping patterns, top nutrition, and great training. This is sexy. This is switched on. This is having A-game. *This* is our well-rounded Alpha.

We are going to cover training for fat loss and muscle building, two key elements in our Alpha's journey. In this we'll cover the training styles outlined above and set out how to attack this over your week.

Everyone has different lives and demands that can raise a few questions about what fit is best for you:

- What level are you currently at?
- How long have you been resistance training? (This is your training age)
- What are your specific goals?
- How do you move?
- What's your daily life like? (Time, workload, stress, energy, nutrition, commitments)
- What is available to you? Are you a gym member? Services of a trainer?

For some people it's easy, for others it's diabolical. So let's agree that regardless of where you are, you need to set aside one hour four times per week initially.

Once your knowledge, strength, and ability grow and you can fine tune your workouts and become efficient with your training time, then perhaps you can decrease this to 45 minutes and then add more sessions if you're capable.

Before we get into the training and what you're going to do there are some fundamentals and crucial points that need addressing and mastering – the nuts and bolts!

Just because you've been lifting weights and been training for a while doesn't mean that you have these basics covered. It also doesn't mean that any workout can't be altered to you. Sometimes the basics are all it takes; just a bit of manipulation of some of our training variables such as weight, tempo, and rest.

For example, if a workout is too easy, decrease your rest or add extra weight. Simple.

Every exercise can be regressed or progressed, depending on your ability or desired outcome, so this is another option.

A barbell squat can be regressed to a dumbbell goblet squat from a seat or progressed by adding weight or a pause at the bottom position. **Always challenge yourself but work within your boundaries.**

Let's run through some quick guidelines:

Always use correct technique and never sacrifice this for weight. Learn to drop the ego and get the load right for the specific movement and parameters.

It defeats the purpose of what you're trying to achieve while increasing the risk/benefit equation. Don't be a hero.

Never train past failure. At times with resistance training, failure is a good thing, causing the right kind of reactions in the body for what we desire. However, trying to push *past* this will more often than not lead to bad form and increase the risk of injury. Until you're highly advanced leave this out.

Always listen to your body and learn to react to how it responds to your training. If something is sore then assess the risk of continuing versus the benefit. On the flip side, if you feel energetic and strong then try another rep or set and do more work!

Also – and this is really important – age is no limit. It might be harder trying to achieve strength and fitness now versus when you were 21 but muscle becomes even more important as we age. Building strong muscles, bones, connective tissue, a strong heart and lungs as well as boosting your testosterone and HGH are crucial to living a long and healthy life. **You're never too old to get strong, lean and muscular!**

The next thing you have to master is training parameters. It's more complicated than lift **X** weight for **X** many times and repeat **X** times. To save us the time of going through tempo, time under tension etc, I've attached this important information to your bonus training start up guide. Check it out, read, absorb, and do.

*** *** ***

While we want to be effective and efficient training beasts you also need to have the right amount of quality rest and recovery to heal, repair, and regenerate your muscles.

You need to be an efficient healer too!

This allows for quicker bounce back from big sessions, less time between big sessions and generally feeling fucking awesome.

Days will come when you're sore, making movement tricky, descending stairs embarrassing, and looking like a duck waddling downhill when walking.

Take note aspiring Alphas – this will happen! You must ensure that to aid recovery you don't just sit still for the day. If you're office and desk bound then as painful as it seems and blatantly feels, get up and move around as often as you can. Those damaged muscles need nutrients to repair and grow and they only get that with nutrient rich blood from the nutrient dense food you've given your body.

This effect known as DOMS – *Delayed Onset Muscle Soreness* – is common, but not always indicative of a good or effective training session. Either way, you need adequate rest.

So besides sleeping, we need some recovery strategies.

Try these recovery strategies on for size:
- Power naps

- Cold showers/ice baths
- Stretching and mobility work
- Remedial massage
- Swimming and water therapy
- Taking full advantage of rest days

Again, see your bonus training guide for in depth tips on the above strategies.

***

Something that can come from poor recovery is an injury. Since injuries suck, this is where being proactive and doing the appropriate mobility and flexibility work comes in. You need to get an idea for what is tight and restricted on your body.

If you can get an assessment from a qualified and experienced trainer or therapist, get them to find what's tight, weak, restricting movement, and what's relatively strong and over active on your body. When we have imbalances we're at increased risk of injury – which we don't want!

Posture is a big part of this and over-training certain muscles is common with guys. It's easy to spot – looking like Quasimodo trying to touch his toes is the more extreme end of this.

As a guideline many men face these common mobility issues:

- Tight thoracic spine
- Poor hip mobility
- Poor ankle mobility
- Tight hip flexors
- Tight chest (pecs) and Lats

(Detailed explanations and remedies in your bonus material)

***

Taking your muscles through the ranges they're designed for will recruit more muscle fibres and therefore get more out of your training. Of course there are times when shorter ranges are appropriate and necessary, but for now we want to hit good range with **perfect technique** – *this is non-negotiable.*

Moving a bar or weight with ugly form may help you get stronger, but not truly strong. Think of it like this – true strength comes as being able to effectively move load with explosive smoothness, awareness of your posture and body in space and control of movement (Rob Williams).

That is to say, when you can move weight with perfect form you're developing real strength and with that comes *real results!* Think of this as your **Physical Intelligence, *your PQ.***

***

Correct technique and moving through proper ranges is a priority, however, there are other key principles for training. Use the following in combination with the other steps in this book and you'll see success.

SIMPLE TRAINING PRINCIPLES

Train often – That doesn't have to be every day but your training days should easily out number your rest days. I mostly run with a 5:2 training:rest ratio. Sure, every little bit helps, but we're about being effective remember – an efficient training beast.

Train hard – Don't fuck around, go balls to the wall and give it your all. The majority of the time when you train, try to do more than last time. This might be faster, heavier, less rest, or simply more overall work. Use your training time wisely and get the most out of it. Use purpose and intensity. People *should* be looking at you if you're putting in enough effort.

Train with purpose – This follows on from above, however, it brings in the element of relative intensity. Training hard isn't always appropriate and sometimes you have to drop it down a gear. However, having purpose to your session is crucial. Don't fall into a trap of "just training"; have a plan, a purpose and knock it off.

Always use perfect form – Be known for your flawless technique. Your strength must be with perfect form and purpose. Increase your PQ. To get truly strong, to quote the ever cheesy infomercial *"It's about technique!"*

Basic lifts come first – This means our primal movement patterns – squat, lunge, bend, push, pull, twist and running (sprinting). Everything else is a combination, regression, or progression of these key movements. These tools alone are enough to turn every man into a beast. Take note in your programs of the patterns with these as a base.

Always aim to do more – This is the concept of progressive overload. Do more work with each workout; be it more reps, weight, sets, or another exercise – even in quicker time. Do more!

If you don't know or are unsure about something, ask – This is as true for the expert as it is for a novice who is learning; asking questions is paramount. Questions provide answers, answers provide results.

Lift heavy and move fast – This means maximal or sub maximal loads. If you're going to get strong, then find your weak points and get cracking. This also means you need to aim to move fast against the weight. Don't just lift it, move it as fast as you can. Focus on activating and squeezing the working muscles.

Sprint like a beast – Sprinting is one of the most basic primal movements and is hands down some of the best training you can do. A hill or stairs is your number one, however, hitting the park or track is just as effective.

Rest, repair and recover – As we've discussed, this is vital for your body to gain the benefits of the hard work you do whilst actually training. Always schedule rest days and make sure you occasionally have a *really* light week of training in order to reset. Always include adequate flexibility and mobility work in order to repair and avoid injury.

Training key point 1: With hypertrophy we're looking to not only increase lean muscle size and volume, but encourage and promote your body to burn fat!

Training key point 2: With strength training we're looking to not only fortify your entire body, but also help toughen your mind. This nervous system training will also act to promote anabolic hormones to get you lean, muscular, and healthy.

Training key point 3: With High Intensity Interval Training (HIIT) we're looking to increase your fitness levels and help improve your cardiovascular and respiratory systems. It's also an amazingly time efficient training tool that promotes fat loss *and muscle building* through the hormonal response. Easily the best bang for your buck cardio exercise, leaving time excuses irrelevant.

Training key point 4: With metabolic resistant training we're looking to produce high output in short times – *hard work*. Promoting fat burning, muscle building, positive hormonal environment, and the beneficial high **Excess Post-exercise Oxygen Consumption** – EPOC.

Training key point 5: One very important thing to remember with weight training is that **there's always a risk. However, we simply make sure that the benefit always outweighs the risk involved.**

Sound easy enough to follow? From here it purely comes down to what to do, which we'll get into shortly and of course actually doing the training. The main thing is to follow those principles. Then, regardless of what actual exercise or training protocol you're following, you'll be getting a great workout and promoting the kind of reactions in your body required to get lean and strong whilst remaining injury free.

Most of the time- Keep it simple, less is more.

THE PROGRAMS
BEAST MODE: PERMANENTLY ON

"Simplicity is the key to brilliance"

- BRUCE LEE

As with your nutrition plans, where you must first master the basics, the same applies for training and lifting – cover the basics mentioned in the simple training philosophies and you'll be on your way to *Alpha-dom – less fat, more muscle, more confidence, more energy, and more sex.*

Now, as a man wanting to shed body fat and increase muscle, if you get a grip on this advice you'll be well on your way. Then, we can integrate some of the specifics. You'll note that throughout this book, these two have mostly been mentioned in tandem, and that's because they don't have to be mutually exclusive. You'll lose body fat and gain lean muscle mass, as well as becoming stronger, fitter, more energetic, and increasing your libido.

However, the number one goal of this plan is to make you look carved from stone. So prepare to do some very hard work. This is where you're going to have to dig deep and find your inner "balls to the wall" attitude and employ it on a regular basis.

To be a real Alpha, you must do the hard yards in your training, or you're simply wasting time.

We're looking to encourage and promote many things to happen inside your body. Here comes your hormones again – this is where the "energy in versus energy out" equation is a bit off.

Yes, we want to burn a lot of energy but as we saw in nutrition, our calories must be quality to begin with. Here it's the same thing – we need quality energy expenditure. Just as different food will trigger different responses in your body, like quality meat promoting insulin sensitivity, so too will the right training trigger the desired hormonal responses that will get you burning fat (and building muscle).

It's important to note that if done effectively, this hormonal activity from training elicits fat burning and muscle building long after the actual training is complete – hence the hours around your training are so important, especially the food you eat, how you rest and how you manage external stressors.

So, when you train to get shredded, it's more than just the training itself – it's more than just the training itself you're after, it's the lasting effects that training creates which are desirable. This is why you need to have purpose, intensity; work your arse off!

This program is split into 3 main phases of 6 weeks, with each phase being split into two separate 3-week phases. In all, you have 18 weeks of training programs and enough training gems to turn you into a beast.

Phase 1: Getting shredded – Greater emphasis on burning fat.

Phase 2: Getting muscular – Focusing more on building muscle. Here, we want to do more of the same in terms of the basics, but we'll be manipulating a few variables, such as, tempo and time under tension to more specifically promote new muscle.

Phase 3: Getting athletic – Focusing on improvements in weak areas. One of the main ones being increased strength, whilst still covering the basics of fat loss and muscle gain.

PHASE 1:
GETTING SHREDDED

You'll see your first 6-week training plan laid over the next few pages. It consists of an initial 3-week phase designed to help build some muscle and increase strength, while still being massively taxing on your system in a way that promotes fast fat burning.

Then you'll move into a second 3-week phase that's less about building muscle and more about marching your fat out the door. This will occur through your intense energy expenditure and immense hormonal manipulation.

Consult your bonus training material to nail down all your training parameters such as tempo and time under tension (TUT), etc.

*Also visit my YouTube channel to see videos of all exercises laid out in the following pages: **youtube.com/user/unleashyouralpha.***

Let's have a look at weeks 1-6; **The Shredded Alpha** phase:

PHASE 1A: WEEKS 1-3

MONDAY	TUESDAY	WEDNESDAY	THURSDAY	FRIDAY	SATURDAY	SUNDAY
WORKOUT A	REST DAY	WORKOUT D	WORKOUT C	REST DAY	WORKOUT B	REST DAY

WORKOUT A

EXERCISE	TUT (S)	TEMPO X-X-X-X	SETS X REPS	REST (S)	ACTUAL LOAD (KG)
A1: Dumbbell goblet squat	40s	3-1-1-0	4 x 8	10s	
A2: Dumbbell walking lunges	60s total	2-0-1-0	4 x 12/leg	10s	
A3: Cable half-kneeling single-arm row	50s/side	3-0-1-0	4 x 12/side	75s	
Rest 2 minutes					
B1: Close supinated grip lat pull down	40s	4-0-1-0	4 x 8	10s	
B2: Cable facepull	50s	3-0-1-1	4 x 10	10s	
B3: Leg press	60s	4-0-1-0	4 x 12	75s	
Rest 2 minutes					
C1: Bodyweight rows	-	Explosive	10-1	-	
C2: Burpees	-	Explosive	10-1	-	

(Complete 10 reps of C1 then 10 of C2 then straight back to 9 reps of each, then 8 and so on down to 1. No rest; as quickly as you can)

WORKOUT B

EXERCISE	TUT (S)	TEMPO X-X-X-X	SETS X REPS	REST (S)	ACTUAL LOAD (KG)
A1: Barbell Romanian dead lift	40s	3-1-1-0	4 x 8	10s	
A2: Swiss ball bent leg hip extension	50s	2-1-1-0	4 x 12	10s	
A3: Cable Paloff press	50s/side	2-0-1-1	4 x 12/ side	75s	
Rest 2 minutes					
B1: Barbell incline press	40s	3-1-1-0	4 x 8	10s	
B2: Dumbbell bench press	50s	3-0-1-1	4 x 10	10s	
B3: Kettlebell/dumbbell dead lift	60s	3-1-1-0	4 x 12	75s	
Rest 2 minutes					
C1: Kettlebell hip swings	-	Explosive	20/18/16 ...2	-	
C2: Medicine ball wallballs	-	Explosive	20/18/16 ...2	-	

(Complete 20 reps of C1 then 20 reps of C2 then straight back to 18 reps of each, then 16, and so on down to 2. No rest; as quickly as you can. Choose a weight for both that's getting tough at 20 for the first round, but you could manage 5-6 more safely)

WORKOUT C

EXERCISE	TUT (S)	REPS/ TIME	ROUNDS	REST (S)	ACTUAL LOAD (KG)
A1: Kettlebell hip swings	-	20 reps	4-5	-	
A2: Rower	-	20 calories	4-5	-	
A3: Standing long jumps	-	30s	4-5	-	
A4: Alternate stepping cable woodchop	-	20 reps (total)	4-5	90-120s	

(Complete exercises A1-A4 as a circuit only resting after A4 for 90-120 seconds, then repeat. Choose weights for A1/A4 that you could do around 25 reps on)

WORKOUT D

EXERCISE	REPS	WORKS (S)	REST (S)
A1: Hill sprints	10-12	20s	60-70s

(Warm up making sure to include some dynamic stretching. Sprint up the hill, ensuring the effort is roughly 20 seconds and at about 85% effort. Walk/jog back down taking note of the rest- keep this standard for now. Repeat for 10-12 reps)

PHASE 1B: WEEKS 4-6

MONDAY	TUESDAY	WEDNESDAY	THURSDAY	FRIDAY	SATURDAY	SUNDAY
REST DAY	WORKOUT B	WORKOUT C	REST DAY	WORKOUT A	WORKOUT D	REST DAY

WORKOUT A

EXERCISE	TUT (S)	TEMPO X-X-X-X	SETS X REPS	REST (S)	ACTUAL LOAD (KG)
A1: Barbell back squat	50s	3-1-1-0	4 x 10	10s	
A2: Dumbbell deficit reverse lunges	60s total	2-0-1-0	4 x 10/leg	10s	
A3: Dumbbell one arm bent over row	50s/side	3-0-1-0	4 x 12/side	60s	
Rest 2 minutes					
B1: (Assisted) chin-ups-neutral grip	40s	3-0-1-0	4 x 10	10s	
B2: Dumbbell pullover	50s	4-0-1-0	4 x 10	10s	
B3: Dumbbell modified cyclist squat	50s	2-0-X-0	4 x 20	60s	
Rest 2 minutes					
C1: Standing long jumps	30s	Explosive	4 x max	None	
C2: Overhead straight-arm med ball slams	30s	Explosive	4 x max	30s	

(Complete 30 seconds of C1 then straight onto 30 seconds of C2, rest 30 seconds and repeat for 4 rounds)

WORKOUT B

EXERCISE	TUT (S)	TEMPO X-X-X-X	SETS X REPS	REST (S)	ACTUAL LOAD (KG)
A1: Dumbbell Romanian Deadlift	45s	3-1-X-0	4 x 10	10s	
A2: Barbell glut bridge	45s	2-0-X-1	4 x 12	10s	
A3: Alternating dumbbell bench press	70s	2-0-1-0	4 x 12/side	60s	
Rest 2 minutes					
B1: (Assisted) Dips	50s	3-1-1-0	4 x 8	10s	
B2: Dumbbell incline press (45°)	50s	3-0-1-0	4 x 12	10s	
B3: Swiss ball hip extension+hamstring curl	60s	2-0-X-0	4 x 12+12	60s	
Rest 2 minutes					
C1: Kettlebell swings	30s	Explosive	4 x 30s	None	
C2: Push-ups	30s	Explosive	4 x 30s	30s	

(Complete 30 seconds of C1 then straight onto 30 seconds of C2, rest 30 seconds and repeat for 4 rounds. Choose a KB weight that 20 reps is starting to be a struggle)

WORKOUT C

EXERCISE	TUT (S)	REPS	ROUNDS	REST (S)	ACTUAL LOAD (KG)
A1: Single-arm squat to press	-	8/10/12/ 10/8	5	-	
A2: Single-arm swing	-	8/10/12/ 10/8	5	-	
A3: Lunge stance row	-	8/10/12/ 10/8	5	-	
A4: Side plank	-	10s/15s/20s/ 15s/10s	5	90s	

(This is a dumbbell complex, so choose one dumbbell. Start on one side and complete 8 reps of A1-A4, and then complete 8 reps of A1-A4 on the other side. Rest 90 seconds and move onto 10 reps per exercise on each side and so on through 12 reps, back to 10 and lastly 8, resting 90 seconds after each full round)

WORKOUT D

EXERCISE	REPS	WORKS (S)	REST (S)
A1: Hill sprints	12-14	20s	50-60s

(Warm up making sure to include some dynamic stretching. Sprint up the hill, ensuring the effort is roughly 20 seconds. Walk/jog back down taking note of the rest – keep this standard for now. Repeat for 10-12 reps)

This program should be hard work, but scale it to suit you. You have a lot of work to cover with little rest so your lungs will scream for oxygen while your muscles will be pumped and burning. These sessions should take around 45 minutes, allowing you some time at the start to do some quick mobility work as a warm up.

The good news is you've now created an environment to stimulate some new muscle while giving your hormones the kick in the arse they need to get you burning fat well into the next day!

You're becoming more Alpha...

PHASE 2:
GETTING MUSCULAR

Don't ever say this again: "I don't want to get big, just defined, you know, *toned.*"

You're here to get massive. Well, *more* massive anyway – it's all relative. What you won't be doing is getting *toned*. This doesn't exist and is such a bad term that not even floppy size-nothing models should use it. You'll be getting muscular from now on, okay?

One of the staples of getting muscular is going to be hypertrophy training. Bodybuilders are the quintessential "muscle gainers," and there have been some amazing ones over the years.

This means actual bona fide competitive bodybuilders, not the guys who think they are by taking every supplement and dropping their weights just to look bad ass.

True body builders are something to admire and respect, especially when you know the insane amount of hard work involved just to put on a few extra kilos of new muscle, let alone become a mountain of a man with a chest that would make a porn star green with envy.

We're definitely promoting the building of new muscle while also getting lean, however, becoming the next Ronnie Coleman is a different book I'm afraid.

***

My approach to gaining muscle is basic yet effective:

- **Lift heavy –** Hypertrophy often calls for relatively lighter weights over longer sets with more reps and less rest than pure strength work. However, moving maximal loads will still stimulate growth due to the immense anabolic response, especially when paired with other lifts and smart nutrition. Also, strengthening your nervous system will cause your muscles to follow suit. If the nervous system isn't getting stronger (through heavy lifting) then your muscles have no pattern to follow.
- **Make sure you change programs regularly, but do not constantly skip from one to the next –** Give your program its due course then make the changes necessary. Anything less and you'll miss out on the gains. Bouncing from one to the next will be detrimental to your results.
- **Move to promote growth –** This may mean hypertrophy, but it also might mean doing some high intensity or sprints sessions to help stimulate your anabolic hormones. Always be stimulating growth, meaning slow cardio is out for now. *Running must be fast.* This goes for lifting too – there are times when a slower pace is needed, but for the most part when you lift a weight, aim to move the weight like your life depends on it!

(This means specifically the 'concentric' phase of the movement – the hard part)

In the workouts below we'll be focusing on the key lifts and complementing them with great muscle building accessory movements while paying attention to the tempo, reps, and rests.

Let's have a look at weeks 7-12; **The Muscular Alpha** phase:

PHASE 2A: WEEKS 7-9

MONDAY	TUESDAY	WEDNESDAY	THURSDAY	FRIDAY	SATURDAY	SUNDAY
WORKOUT C	WORKOUT A	REST DAY	WORKOUT D	REST DAY	WORKOUT B	REST DAY

WORKOUT A

EXERCISE	TUT (S)	TEMPO X-X-X-X	SETS X REPS	REST (S)	ACTUAL LOAD (KG)
A: Supinated grip chin-ups	25-30s	4-0-X-0	4 x 6	75s	
Rest 2 minutes					
B1: Dumbbell seated overhead press (45° semi-pronated grip)	50s	4-0-1-0	4 x 10	60s	
B2: Single-arm lat pulldown	40s/side	3-0-1-0	4 x 10/ side	60s	
Rest 2 minutes					
C1: Barbell incline press (medium grip)	50s	3-1-1-0	4 x 10	45s	
C2: Dumbbell incline curl (supinated)	50s	3-0-1-1	4 x 10	45s	

WORKOUT B

EXERCISE	TUT (S)	TEMPO X-X-X-X	SETS X REPS	REST (S)	ACTUAL LOAD (KG)
A: Close-grip bench press	25-30s	4-0-X-0	4 x 6	75s	
Rest 2 minutes					
B1: Weighted push-ups	50s	3-0-1-1	4 x 10	60s	
B2: Wide-grip seated row	50s	3-0-1-1	4 x 10	60s	
Rest 2 minutes					
C1: Decline EZ bar skullcrushers	50s	3-0-1-1	4 x 10	45s	
C2: Cable modified face pull	60s	3-0-1-1	4 x 12	45s	

WORKOUT C

EXERCISE	TUT (S)	TEMPO X-X-X-X	SETS X REPS	REST (S)	ACTUAL LOAD (KG)
A: Barbell back squat	25-30s	3-1-X-0	4 x 6	75s	
Rest 2 minutes					
B1: Dumbbell walking lunge	50s	2-0-X-0	4 x 10/leg	60s	
B2: Barbell good morning	45s	4-0-X-0	4 x 10	60s	
Rest 2 minutes					
C1: Dumbbell modified cyclist squat	50s	2-0-X-0	4 x 20	45s	
C2: Hyperextensions	50s	4-0-1-0	4 x 10	45s	

WORKOUT D

EXERCISE	TUT (S)	TEMPO X-X-X-X	SETS X REPS	REST (S)	ACTUAL LOAD (KG)
A: Barbell Romanian deadlift	25-30s	4-0-X-0	4 x 6	75s	
Rest 2 minutes					
B1: Barbell glut bridge	45s	2-1-X-1	4 x 10	60s	
B2: Dumbbell deficit reverse lunge	50s	2-0-X-0	4 x 10/leg	60s	
Rest 2 minutes					
C1: Kettlebell hip swings (heavy)	20s	Explosive	4 x 10	10s	
C2: Leg press	50s	4-0-1-0	4 x 10	45s	

(Kettlebell swings in this example are heavy – 10 tough reps!)

PHASE 2B: WEEKS 10-12

MONDAY	TUESDAY	WEDNESDAY	THURSDAY	FRIDAY	SATURDAY	SUNDAY
WORKOUT D	WORKOUT B	WORKOUT E	REST DAY	WORKOUT C	WORKOUT A	REST DAY

You'll see that this phase has taken a step up in volume *and* intensity. So strap your hard pants on and unleash your inner beast. There's no soft way through this phase.

WORKOUT A

EXERCISE	TUT (S)	TEMPO X-X-X-X	SETS X REPS	REST (S)	ACTUAL LOAD (KG)
A: Neutral grip chin-ups	35s	4-0-X-0	4 x 8	75s	
Rest 2 minutes					
B1: Lat pulldown-pronated grip	50s	3-0-1-1	4 x 10	60s	
B2: Dumbbell seated Arnold press	50s	4-0-1-0	4 x 10	60s	
Rest 2 minutes					
C1: EZ bar preacher curl	60s	3-0-1-1	3 x 12	45s	
C2: Barbell incline press-wide grip	60s	3-1-1-0	3 x 10	45s	
Rest 2 minutes					
D: Supinated chin-ups	5 mins density- Do as many reps as you can in 5 minutes				

(Rest when needed but as little as possible, and complete as many full, quality reps as you can in the 5 minutes. Take note and aim to do more each week)

WORKOUT B

EXERCISE	TUT (S)	TEMPO X-X-X-X	SETS X REPS	REST (S)	ACTUAL LOAD (KG)
A: Medium grip bench press	45s	3-1-X-1	4 x 8	75s	
Rest 2 minutes					
B1: Close-grip push-ups	45s	3-1-X-0	4 x 10	60s	
B2: Dumbbell one-arm bent over row	40s	3-0-1-0	4 x 10	60s	
Rest 2 minutes					
C1: Dumbbell skull crushers	60s	3-1-1-0	3 x 12	45s	
C2: Cable facepull	60s	3-1-1-0	3 x 10	45s	
Rest 2 minutes					
D: Dumbbell chest press	Rest-pause: 3 sets, 30s rest, 2-0-X-0 tempo with 10RM weight				

(Complete 8 reps of your 10RM weight on the dumbbell press, rest 30 seconds and then complete as many reps as you can. Rest another 30 seconds and complete as many reps as you can again – that's it)

WORKOUT C

EXERCISE	TUT (S)	TEMPO X-X-X-X	SETS X REPS	REST (S)	ACTUAL LOAD (KG)
A: Barbell back squat	40s	4-0-1-0	4 x 8	75s	
Rest 2 minutes					
B1: Barbell walking lunge	70s total	2-1-X-0	4 x 10/leg	60s	
B2: Hyperextensions	45s	3-1-X-0	4 x 10	60s	
Rest 2 minutes					
C1: Dumbbell modified cyclist 1 & 1/4 squat	60s	2-0-X-0	3 x 15	45s	
C2: Barbell good morning	60s	4-0-X-0	3 x 12	45s	
Rest 2 minutes					
D: Sled push/pull	4 mins of 20s on/10s off				

(This should be balls to the wall brutal. If you don't have access to a sled or Prowler you can push a car (seriously) or do treadmill incline sprints instead. Sprint on an incline set about 7% for 20s then jump off to the side while the belt still spins. Rest 10s then jump back on and go again – 8 rounds)

WORKOUT D

EXERCISE	TUT (S)	TEMPO X-X-X-X	SETS X REPS	REST (S)	ACTUAL LOAD (KG)
A: Barbell deadlift	40s	3-0-X-0	4 x 8	75s	
Rest 2 minutes					
B1: Dumbbell side lunge	50s total	2-0-X-0	4 x 10/leg	60s	
B2: Dumbbell step-up	60s total	2-0-1 -0	4 x 10/leg	60s	
Rest 2 minutes					
C1: Kettlebell swings (heavy)	20s	Explosive	3 x 12	45s	
C2: Leg press- toes out	60s	4-0-1-0	3 x 12	45s	
Rest 2 minutes					
D: Trap-bar dead lift	Rest-pause: 3 sets, 20s rest, 2-0-X-0 tempo with 10RM weight				

(Complete 8 reps of your 10RM weight on the dumbbell press, rest 20 seconds and then complete as many reps as you can. Rest another 20 seconds and complete as many reps as you can again – that's it.)

WORKOUT E

EXERCISE	REPS	WORKS (S)	REST (S)
A1: Hill sprints	10-12	30s	90s

(Warm up making sure to include some dynamic stretching. Sprint up the hill, ensuring the effort is roughly 30 seconds. Walk/jog back down so you're ready to go again after 90s seconds rest – each effort should start on 2 minutes. Repeat for 10-12 reps)

As you can see there's a bit to get through but all the information's there to get you smashing through these workouts, building muscle, and cursing my name for creating it. Make sure you stick to the tempos and TUT. This program will tear and create new muscle whist also getting your hormones peaking to turn you into a lean and jacked Alpha.

Check out your bonus training tips for a bunch of extra muscle building gems.

"Everybody wanna be a body builder, don't nobody want to lift no god damn heavy-ass weights!"

- 8 TIME MR OLYMPIA RONNIE COLEMAN

PHASE 3:
GETTING ATHLETIC

Start thinking and treating yourself like an athlete – prioritise sleep, fun, health, eating well, and looking good. Once you've done the hard work from the previous pages, you'll be at a point where tinkering your training to that of a bona fide athlete is simple and provides endless options.

Becoming truly strong for your shape, weight, and height is no mean feat and is a real challenge for any man. So the tests and work involved to move maximal loads at speed is a great discipline. There is the obvious benefit of increasing strength, however, your hormones are still very much at play here.

Let's have a look at weeks 13-18; *The Athletic Alpha* phase:

PHASE 3A: WEEKS 13-15

MONDAY	TUESDAY	WEDNESDAY	THURSDAY	FRIDAY	SATURDAY	SUNDAY
WORKOUT C	WORKOUT A	WORKOUT E	REST DAY	WORKOUT D	WORKOUT B	REST DAY

WORKOUT A

EXERCISE	TUT (S)	TEMPO X-X-X-X	SETS X REPS	REST (S)	ACTUAL LOAD (KG)
A: Supinated grip chin-ups	18s	3-0-X-0	5 x 5	90s	
Rest 2 minutes					
B1: Barbell military press	40s	4-0-X-0	4 x 8	75s	
B2: Dumbbell one-arm bent over row	40s/side	3-1-X-0	4 x 8/side	75s	
Rest 2 minutes					
C1: Supine bodyweight row	-	Explosive	10-1	-	
C2: Dumbbell push press	-	Explosive	10-1	-	

(Complete 10 reps of C1 then 10 of C2 and then straight back to 9 reps of each, then 8 and so on down to 1. No rest, as quickly as you can. Pick a weight for the push press that you could safely complete an 11th or maybe 12th rep to start)

WORKOUT B

EXERCISE	TUT (S)	TEMPO X-X-X-X	SETS X REPS	REST (S)	ACTUAL LOAD (KG)
A: Medium grip bench press	18s	3-0-X-0	5 x 5	90s	
Rest 2 minutes					
B1: Dips	40s	3-1-X-0	4 x 8	75s	
B2: Lat pulldown, pronated	40s	3-1-X-0	4 x 8	75s	
Rest 2 minutes					
C1: Push-ups	-	Explosive	Max	-	
C2: Straight-arm med ball slams	-	Explosive	20	45s	

(Complete as many reps of C1 as you can and then move to C2, then rest for 45 seconds and repeat for 4 rounds. Aim to get at least 15-20 push-ups, so if you struggle after a set or two, bring your hands up off the ground onto a bench or similar so you're on an incline)

WORKOUT C

EXERCISE	TUT (S)	TEMPO X-X-X-X	SETS X REPS	REST (S)	ACTUAL LOAD (KG)
A: Barbell deadlift	12s	2-0-X-0	5 x 5	90s	
Rest 2 minutes					
B1: Barbell front squat	40s	3-1-X-0	4 x 8	75s	
B2: Hyperextensions	40s	4-0-X-0	4 x 8	75s	
Rest 2 minutes					
C1: Kettlebell swings	30s	Explosive	20	-	
C2: Standing long jumps	30s	Explosive	30s	45-60s	

(Complete 20 reps of C1 as fast as you can and then move to C2 for as many reps as you can in 30 seconds, then rest for 45 seconds and repeat for 4 rounds. Swings are lighter so you can complete 20 reps, but still ensure they're heavy enough to engage a powerful hip drive on the last few reps. Have a bit more rest if needed)

WORKOUT D

EXERCISE	TUT (S)	TEMPO X-X-X-X	SETS X REPS	REST (S)	ACTUAL LOAD (KG)
A: Barbell back squat	18s	3-0-X-0	5 x 5	90s	
Rest 2 minutes					
B1: Barbell good morning	35s	3-0-X-0	4 x 8	75s	
B2: Dumbbell side lunge	20s/leg	2-0-X-0	4 x 8/leg	75s	
Rest 2 minutes					
D: Trap-bar dead lift (8-10RM)	5 mins density- do as many reps as you can in 5 minutes				

(Rest as needed but as little as possible and complete as many full, quality reps as you can in the 5 minutes. For this pick a weight that would be around your 10 rep max, but not heavier. We still want a strength element to this. If you can get more than 50 it's too light; if you can only get 20-30 it's too heavy.)

WORKOUT E

EXERCISE	REPS	WORKS (S)	REST (S)
A1: Rower interval sprints	10	30s	30s

(Warm-up making sure to include some dynamic stretching. Set the rower to interval with 30 seconds work : 30 seconds rest. Try to stay consistent throughout the 10 rounds with your effort and distance covered. This is short but sharp and should have you hating life temporarily at the end)

PHASE 3B: WEEKS 16-18

MONDAY	TUESDAY	WEDNESDAY	THURSDAY	FRIDAY	SATURDAY	SUNDAY
WORKOUT C	WORKOUT A	WORKOUT E	REST DAY	WORKOUT D	WORKOUT B	REST DAY

WORKOUT A

EXERCISE	TUT (S)	TEMPO X-X-X-X	SETS X REPS	REST (S)	ACTUAL LOAD (KG)
A: Neutral grip chin-ups	15s	3-0-X-0	6 x 4	90s	
Rest 2 minutes					
B: Dumbbell bench press	10 mins density – as many reps as you can in 10 minutes, 2-0-X-0, rest as needed, 10RM weight				
Rest 2 minutes					
C1: Supinated chin-ups	-	Explosive	10-1	As needed	
C2: Push-ups	-	Explosive	1-10	As needed	

(Complete 10 reps of C1 then 1 of C2, then straight back to 9 reps of C1 and 2 reps of C2, then 8 of C1 and 3 of C2 and so on down to until they criss-cross and you do 1 rep of C1 and 10 of C2. As little rest as possible; complete as quickly as you can and make sure you time it so you can improve each time)

WORKOUT B

EXERCISE	TUT (S)	TEMPO X-X-X-X	SETS X REPS	REST (S)	ACTUAL LOAD (KG)
A: Barbell incline press-medium grip	15s	3-0-X-0	6 x 4	90s	
Rest 2 minutes					
B: Dumbbell one-arm bent over row	10 mins density – as many reps as you can evenly on both sides in 10 minutes, 2-0-X-0, rest as needed, 10RM weight				
Rest 2 minutes					
C1: Dips	-	2-0-X-0	Max	-	
C2: Farmer's carry	30s	-	30s walk	45s	

(Complete as many reps of C1 as you can, then pick up two heavy kettlebells or dumbbells and walk for 30 seconds, then rest for 45 seconds and repeat for 4 rounds)

WORKOUT C

EXERCISE	TUT (S)	TEMPO X-X-X-X	SETS X REPS	REST (S)	ACTUAL LOAD (KG)
A: Barbell sumo deadlift	10s	2-0-X-0	6 x 4	90s	
Rest 2 minutes					
B: Barbell front squat	10 mins density – as many reps as you can in 10 minutes, 2-0-X-0, rest as needed, 10RM weight				
Rest 2 minutes					
C1: Kettlebell swings (heavy)	20s	Explosive	4 x 12	-	
C2: Box jumps (high)	30s	Explosive	4 x 20	60-90s	

(The swings might mean using two dumbbells or one large dumbbell to get a heavy enough weight. Make box jumps high enough that you have to explode off the ground to get up. Aim for 60s rest but extend to 90s if necessary)

WORKOUT D

EXERCISE	TUT (S)	TEMPO X-X-X-X	SETS X REPS	REST (S)	ACTUAL LOAD (KG)
A: Barbell back squat	15s	3-0-X-0	6 x 4	90s	
Rest 2 minutes					
B: Trap-bar dead lift	10 mins density – as many reps as you can in 10 minutes, 2-0-X-0, rest as needed, 8-10RM weight				
Rest 2 minutes					
C: Sled drags	30s	Explosive	5 rounds	30s	

(This should be balls to the wall brutal. If you don't have access to a sled or Prowler you can push a car – seriously – or hill sprints on the treadmill- 30s on/30s off, 6-8 reps)

WORKOUT E

EXERCISE	REPS	WORKS (S)	REST (S)
A1: Hill sprints	12-14	20s	40s

(Warm-up making sure to include some dynamic stretching. Sprint up the hill, ensuring the effort is roughly 20 seconds. Walk/jog back down so you start every effort on 60 seconds. Repeat for 10-12 reps)

Note that the same principles can be applied to the man on holiday or travelling for work and has limited time and resources. In your bonus training tips material you'll find all the details and best tips for training while on holiday or on work trips away.

As with nutrition, there are different ways to train and different methodologies. However, our aim is to keep things simple, take the confusion out and get you lean, muscular, and developing your athletic A-game. What we've covered is the information to do just that, it's up to you now to implement and start kicking some serious arse.

You now have the tools to train for shredded fat loss, to put on serious muscular size, *and* to increase your strength.

As you already know, to put on new muscle and become a lean beast, you have to balance the other areas of your life and get them working in unison with each other.

Think of it like this – **if you train for 4 hours per week, that's 4 hours out of a 168-hour week – a very small proportion.**

What you do for those other 162 hours is monumental! Sleep will be a big part of it, but you'll also eat, work, move, stress, relax, and just be *you* – the more you can get the rest of those hours to line up with the monster work you're doing in the gym, the better your results will be. Not only this, but the habitual changes that become a part of it will make this much easier to maintain long term, which is the key to being a true Alpha!

* *Keep reading on and check out the **Unleash Your Alpha case studies with Will and Drew** to see how following the training protocols laid out on the previous pages not only turned their bodies around, but helped to stimulate great changes in their lives too.*

JUST RELAX

BALANCE – HOW TO MASTER SLEEP, STRESS AND ENJOY YOUR LIFE

"Most men die at 25… we just don't bury them until they are 70."

- BENJAMIN FRANKLIN

It seems like a stupidly obvious thing to say: *life is for living*. What else are we doing here if we're not living? Well, it does make you think – if we're not living then are we simply dying? Perhaps more apt, are we just wasting time until we die?

This is the case for so many. A common example is the man who gets up each morning after hitting snooze a couple of times – it dawns on him (or doesn't, even worse) that he's about to embark on another unfruitful day of moving from A to B and going through the same familiar motions that he does every day. Except for the weekend, which he absolutely lives for because the week contains so much stress and so little time and enjoyment that he longs for it. Then the weekend passes like a flash of lightning in the dark night and he's back hitting snooze again to heavy tired eyes come Monday morning. Again.

Mediocrity at its infinite, repetitive, and frightfully common best. Whatever happened to striving for more? Never being satisfied? Doing what makes you happy? Creating a life that you love and generating enjoyment from every day?

The road out is multifaceted, however, it needn't be so complex. We've looked at *thought, nutrition, and training.* Now, how we approach and manage our sleep, stress, and enjoyment are vital to living a great life, but also what state your mind *and* body will be in.

This may sound like an extreme case but it's not. With adequate rest, sleep, stress levels, and a more positive outlook this man can change things and turn it around.

However, without that change, all the exercise, great food, and determination won't do it. Conditions such as adrenal fatigue are very common these days, which often goes undiagnosed in many people. This will cause a cascade of negative effects from body composition worsening, energy dropping, mood declining, and illness a constant threat.

Are you starting to see just how connected all of this stuff is and how each element is as crucial as the next? Of course some will hold more importance at times and depending on the man. However, each component must be a well-oiled cog in the wheel of your life in order for you to become a true Alpha and find your A-game.

Just like you are with your food and drink, start keeping a diary of your sleep, stress, and enjoyment levels. You'll find your diary with your bonus material – start on it today. Record specific details, stress triggers, what you enjoyed that day – anything you think is relevant. The form will guide you.

In order for you to make some real progress in this area you must first realise what's happening and where your strengths and weaknesses are so you can use the appropriate strategies where needed.

Life is for living, not existing.

SLEEP

"Sleep is God. Go worship."

- JIM BUTCHER

Some people love it and value it so highly they schedule power naps into their day, others have a more dysfunctional relationship with life's innate healer. There's a reason we can't go very long without sleep – **we'll die!** On a lesser scale, without adequate quality sleep we'll function poorly and open ourselves up to illness or "lesser death".

One of the best tools for turning Alpha is getting enough quality sleep. This is sadly underrated and is why Western society has so many stressed out, overweight, and hormonally screwed men.

Sleep has long been thought of as a function to give the brain rest, of which it undoubtedly does. Fatigue, symptomatic of reduced cognitive ability and decreased alertness are glaring obvious with a lack of sleep. However, sleep also functions to regulate hormones that affect energy production and use. Sleep also affects body composition and risk of various diseases such as diabetes.

One study showed this in a comprehensive fashion. A team

of researchers at the *University Of Chicago Medicine* found that while many people claim to handle the cognitive effects of routine sleep deprivation, they weren't tolerating the metabolic and physiological consequences.

This study, published in the *Annals of Internal Medicine* was thoroughly carried out and examined the insulin response in young, lean, and healthy subjects who went through two different study conditions – 8.5 hours sleep per night and 4.5 hours sleep per night both for 4 consecutive nights, with food intake controlled under both conditions.

The researchers found that overall body response to insulin dropped by an average 16% and fat cell insulin sensitivity decreased by 30% when the participants were sleep deprived. The authors stated, "When fat cells cannot respond effectively to insulin, these lipids leach out into the circulation, leading to serious complications." We've seen this earlier in fat gain with the risk of illness and serious chronic diseases like diabetes and heart disease.

Again, this comes back to hormonal control and regulation. Getting enough quality sleep is entirely dependent on your hormonal activity, and the components of your daily life affect this. What this means is that you *can* have a profound effect on your health and body composition by sorting your sleeping out.

The other major action and benefit of adequate sleep is healing and recovery. This will obviously encourage desirable hormonal activity (as we saw earlier with HGH) but it will also help to specifically repair tissue that's injured and damaged.

This is a huge requirement of the hard training man. Great sleep will help to repair inflamed tissue from many life stressors including exercise. Great sleep will also help to reduce oxidative stress and its negative effects on the body, whilst also aiding the liver and kidneys to do their job in keeping you healthy.

These are very common issues, and heavy training will increase these risks, hence why diet and adequate rest are so imperative to ensure recovery from the hard work you do.

Outside of just plain getting more sleep and prioritising it more highly in your life, there are many things you can do to get *more* sleep, get *better quality* sleep, and make sure you wake each day feeling *fresh* and ready to kick goals.

LIFE BALANCE STRATEGY 1: SLEEPING STRATEGIES

Let's look at some great strategies to help you improve your sleep habits. *Aim to get at least 7 hours of deep restful sleep, but no more than 9, each night.*

Switch off – We live in a busy world that's constantly grabbing our attention. Whether it's work, family, technology or our own minds, we're relentlessly bombarded by stressor after stressor and one demand for our attention after another.

This affects our mind and eventually our hormones, with cortisol increase a direct response to increased stress. This will heavily affect your ability to both fall asleep and have a great deep sleep. So, for that to decrease, you have to switch off sufficiently each night and wind your mind down to promote your parasympathetic nervous system in order for "rest and digest" to ensue.

Here are some great tactics to switch off:

- **Install light altering software on your computer to adapt to time of day –** As you'll see below this light isn't good at night, but you can also get a jump on it by installing software that will dim and adjust the light according to the time of day. Try http://stereopsis.com/flux/ for your free download.

- **Do not watch or look at electronics at least 30 minutes before bed -** That means TV, computer, and smart phones. The blue light from these excite your pineal gland, which will stimulate you in a way that causes you to stay awake longer.
- **Dim the lights in the hour before bed –** Same thing, start reminding the body and brain that sleep time is approaching. Having bright lights shining until you get into bed discourages your body's natural sleep clock and production of melatonin, which is necessary to regulate sleeping (as well as crucial brain functions and immune system support).
- **Remove electronics from the bedroom –** This will not only prevent random stimulation in the form of annoying mates waking you in the middle of the night with a text, but as seen above, these devices act to disrupt the pineal gland.
- **No work at least 30 minutes prior to bed –** This means avoiding anything that stimulates your mind, so anything mildly intellectual. This window must be for relaxing and winding down.
- **Brain dump –** If you often struggle to unwind and switch off because you have the day's brain activity wildly moving you from thought to thought and preventing your mind from relaxing, then a brain dump before bed can work wonders. Simply get a pad and pen and get writing. Set a timer for 10 minutes and get it all out. Your gratitude journal works wonders here as well.

- **Read something mindless –** This should be light and entertaining (even boring) as opposed to anything that gets your mind thinking and stimulated.
- **Meditate –** This isn't for everyone, but it can work wonders to down regulate your brain activity and leave you in a chilled state. This doesn't have to be meditation in the traditional sense of the word, it can simply be focusing your mind on something in particular and really being in that moment. Stare at the wall if you like. Also, try downloading a sleep meditation podcast. This kind of sound frequency will aid in switching off your brain until you're more skilled at it. Electronics are okay in the short term for this purpose.
- **Level your breathing and heart rate –** It may sound painfully obvious, but breathing is vital to proper sleep. Most people don't breathe using their diaphragm, which leads to a host of dysfunction. To really control your heart rate and help you switch off when in bed, practise taking deep diaphragmatic breaths. Place a hand on your stomach and inhale as large as you can through your nose. Your stomach should move out long before your chest expands. Exhale long and slow as you draw your stomach back in. Repeat 10 times.
- **Shower –** Besides getting the day's grime off you before getting into your sheets, showering can help to wind you down and switch off. I recommend having a cold shower; this will force you to control your breathing and help your mind exit anything else that would prevent you from sleeping.
  Challenge Give it a go for 2 weeks – begin by starting your shower on cold for 30 seconds and progress until you have the entire length of the shower on cold. This

will also act as a form of meditation if you can focus on the sensation of the water hitting your body and levelling your breathing. Studies have shown cold therapy like this to have numerous health benefits also.

Don't sleep in late – Waking at 8am will invariably mean one or two things – you're sleeping too long or staying up too late. Waking this late will trick your body into thinking bed time is very far away, so after a hectic day of Alpha activity when it comes time to sleep, your subconscious may think differently. Get up before 7 at the latest; then not only will you be able to regulate this pattern better, but also you'll get more done!

Go to bed earlier – This may sound like beating a broken record into submission, but going to bed late is detrimental to regular sleeping patterns. If it's because you aren't tired then you might need to up your energy output; if it's because you're "too busy" then go back to your values and goals and see what you really want. If it's anything to do with your body and being more awesome (or any of the success points we've covered) then prioritise getting a better night's sleep over working until stupid o'clock. *Seriously.*

Train earlier in the day – If you can only find the time to train after work then the effects of this workout may be preventing you from nodding off. Try to reorganise your day and get your training in earlier.

Get some sun/Vitamin D – Not only is regular sun exposure crucial for adequate vitamin D and its health benefits but it will help your melatonin production, which is your natural sleep hormone.

Have sex – Besides the fact you're acting on man's most primal urge, sex is a great sign of testosterone and health. It will also tire you out and do its best to sedate you. Short and sharp is best for sending you off to sleep – no long duration cardio sessions. Also, your testosterone peaks in the morning, so if you wake with a full mast (and it's plausible) then have sex. This surge of testosterone will help in everything we're trying to achieve.

Eat earlier in the night – If you're getting home late and eating not long before bed this could be causing you to stay awake as your body is actively digesting when you're trying to drop off.

Eat carbs at night – On days that you train, choose good quality carb options for your last meal of the day which will help boost melatonin. Not only this, but having these carb options, such as sweet potato, beet root or quinoa at night, will provide you with great energy for the morning especially if that's when you train.

Do something that makes you happy – This seems like a "goes without saying" strategy, however, so many men go to bed either stressed and unhappy, or already thinking about the dread the following day brings. Find something you enjoy, without electronics, (see above) and do it. Walk along the beach if you live close to it, call a close friend and chat for 10 minutes, read that vintage *Penthouse Forum* you have from back in the day. Whatever it is, do it.

Get in a power nap – This isn't necessarily a realistic strategy for many, however, if it's possible try getting in a power nap. Aim for no longer than 30 minutes; sometimes as little as 5-10 minutes will suffice.

Supplement with magnesium, zinc & Vitamin B6 or ZMA – As seen in your bonus supplementation material, these individual or combined substances are crucial for repair and healing while also aiding you to drop off into a deep, restful sleep.

Do your nightly rituals after dinner – If you normally floss and brush your teeth before going to bed, or perhaps put the trash out, do it well before bedtime. If your body feels like it's time for bed but you stall that by going about a set of chores or routines, you're messing with your natural urge to sleep. Get these things out of the way so when bedtime arrives you can simply get in and go to sleep.

Use a sleep app – This can be extremely useful in monitoring sleeping patterns. Use it to get a picture of your sleep, including, average hours/night and overall quality – deep or shallow. Try for 2-3 months then go back to removing your phone from your room. Make sure you put your phone on flight mode (do this if it's also your alarm clock).

Enjoy sleep – One thing that affects so many men is stressing over sleep. This only exacerbates the problem, acting to increase cortisol and decrease your chances of a decent night's sleep. Learn to enjoy sleep and know that with the above strategies in place, you'll be getting off to a quality sleep in no time.

This list should give you enough workable and effective strategies to enable you to fall asleep quicker, sleep better, and wake feeling refreshed and ready to crack into the day ahead. Not all strategies will work or be appropriate for you, but experiment and see what does. At a minimum, put the necessary steps in place to get consistently great sleep.

STRESS AND ENJOYING LIFE

"The moment you stop doing things for fun, you may as well be dead"

- ERNEST HEMMINGWAY

We've seen how interrelated our hormones are. They're complex and dependent on one another as well as any number of lifestyle factors such as food, training, and definitely sleep. However, they don't need to be too complicated – and when it comes to healing, burning fat, growing muscle, getting a good night's sleep, and being healthy, we have the steps and strategies laid out so far. Now one of other main contributors that hold many men back is stress. More specifically, too damn much of it!

As we've seen, operating in a constant or even semi-constant, state of "fight or flight" will cause your body to become inflamed, have high levels of oxidative stress, store fat, and always be on the ready, waiting for some big stressor. On a biological level your body is readying for attack or survival. Long term this is terrible for you, your health and any Alpha aspirations. Your body will will hate you for it.

The saying "stress kills" isn't just to ward off high achieving, pushy, and unrealistic bosses – it's because the effects *will kill you*.

Unnecessary stress is the main contributor to high cortisol levels and the cycle that comes from poor sleep, body fat gain, and general poor health. So, we must manage this stress to gain from all the hard work you'll be doing everywhere else.

You're also at the risk of *adrenal fatigue*. This occurs when the adrenal glands become exhausted, overworked, and unable to handle the continuous demands of constant SNS activity.

The kind of triggers that can affect the adrenal glands in this way are: high levels of stress, anger, fear, anxiety, guilt, depression, overwork, excessive exercise, sleep deprivation, light-cycle disruption (such as working the night shift, often going to sleep late or regularly crossing time zones), surgery, trauma or injury, chronic inflammation, infection, illness or pain, temperature extremes, toxic exposure, nutritional deficiencies and/or severe allergies.

Common signs and symptoms may include:

- Fatigue and weakness, especially in the morning and afternoon
- A suppressed immune system
- Increased allergies
- Muscle and bone loss and muscular weakness
- Depression
- Cravings for foods high in salt, sugar or fat
- Hormonal imbalance (*we already know this is happening*)
- Skin problems
- Autoimmune disorders
- Low sex drive
- Light-headedness when getting up from sitting or lying down
- Decreased ability to handle stress

- Trouble waking up in the morning, despite a full night's sleep
- Poor memory

In some more severe cases sufferers may find it hard to even get out of bed. Now this may sound a long way off, but if early signs are left to develop and worsen this can lead to anywhere from 9-24 months recovery.

It's absolutely imperative that stress and stressors are managed appropriately.

In his book *Adrenal Fatigue: The 21st Century Stress Syndrome*, James Wilson estimates that around 80% of all adults experience some level of adrenal fatigue in their lifetimes. However, it largely goes undiagnosed by modern medicine, therefore becoming an increasingly influential player in the health and lives of us men.

You now know the importance of our hormones – your adrenal glands secrete more than 50 hormones! So if they aren't functioning properly, *you* aren't functioning properly. You can forget about burning fat or putting on lean muscle, and worry more about having the energy to get through the day without feeling like shit, or more specifically, without crucial bodily functions such as the regulation of metabolic function, blood sugar levels, and sex hormones.

***

Some of the best strategies to manage short-term stress are the ones we went through in the prior the sleep work, in particular:

- **Switch off** (brain dump, reading mindless material, meditation of some form, breathing control, cold shower)

- **Have sex**
- **Do something you enjoy**

This last one is the clincher and the obvious part of de-stressing. Definitely use these tactics in combination – try to clear your mind and leave work at work, not bring it home, especially to bed. However, we're going to have a closer look at doing things that you enjoy and make you grow.

Before you set off with this you need to take stock of what has been stressing you out, how you've been handling it and what you've been enjoying out of each day. Go to your stress diary and see what the specifics are. Also, note the things you enjoy that have been missing, as these are some of the things you need to implement into your life.

First, let's look back at your thoughts earlier on – are you happy? What do you value in life the most? What is your approach to life like?

We're trying to promote a positive mindset every day. This isn't to say you won't have tough moments, days, even months, but you need to start doing things that make you happy and that help you grow and get closer to what your real passion in life is. Go back to your goals, values, and passion. See where these fit in your current life and think seriously about the why and how to get there. Then you can implement the below strategies to *de-stress long term*.

As we saw earlier with your 'physical intelligence', now we are also wanting to work on and improve your emotional intelligence and your spiritual intelligence.

LIFE BALANCE STRATEGY 2: STRATEGIES FOR LONG TERM STRESS MANAGEMENT THROUGH ENJOYMENT AND POSITIVITY:

Mindset – As discussed above, this is where it starts. Long-term stress management depends on a positive attitude and open mind. Get specific with what you value and go in search of it.

Get centred – This could be simple meditation that you schedule on a daily basis. However, if you need some calm immediately then learning to "centre yourself" can be amazingly effective. The main thing is to *just be in the moment*. Empty your mind of all distractions and negative thoughts. Focus on something that you wouldn't normally feel, such as the feel of your feet in your shoes, or the wind on your face. Stop, focus, and *really* feel it. Listen to the sounds, smell the air. If done properly, this will be enough to clear you mind and reset your nervous system to a more parasympathetic state.

Practice gratitude in shitty moments – When you get angry or pissed off at something small, try self managing this by pulling your head in and practising gratitude. Stop, think of two things you're grateful for and change your state of mind – get out of the funk.

Comfort zone breakers – Your comfort zone is nice and cosy and warm. It's also holding you back. When you get out beyond yourself you'll not only start to become happier, you'll better yourself and unleash your inner Alpha. A true Alpha lives outside his comfort zone and is constantly improving himself. Start doing things that make you uncomfortable, therefore out of your precious zone. It doesn't have to be huge, but everyday things. Of course in saying that it can also be something that scares the living shit out of you. Let's look at some examples:

- **Fill out and *share* your goals, values, mission and 5-year visualisation –** This is usually way outside the comfort zone of many guys, so start by putting 100% effort into this task.
- **Set one massive and well over-the-top long term goal –** This could be anything, for example mine for 2012 was to source, cook, and eat a different meat *every* week for the entire year – 52 meats – and blogged about it. This took me outside of my comfort zone almost weekly.
- **Call someone you've been meaning to call, but been avoiding it –** Simple little tasks like this are easy little daily ways to break the zone.
- **Cook something for someone that you've never even eaten –** Never eaten lamb's balls before? Get some fresh balls and cook them for someone else. This should make you uncomfortable enough for one evening! The reward and growth could be huge, or, try something a little less testicle to start with.
- **Eat something you've never tried and always avoided –** Sometimes as children we "decide" we don't like eating something even without trying it. Plus as you grow your tastes change. Pick one and eat it. For me this was onions – I swore I would never eat them knowingly – now I *choose* to cook with them.
- **If you're a tight arse go splurge and vice versa –** If you never spend money on things you consider unnecessary then find something you'd love but don't need and splurge on it. If you always spend money on things you potentially don't *need* then stop yourself from making those next three purchases.

- **Tell someone your most personal goal –** This will act to add serious accountability to your goal.
- **Don't touch alcohol for an entire month –** Besides the obvious health benefits, this is usually something most guys find extremely difficult, so do it at a tough time, say Christmas or on holiday. The peer pressure alone will make you pine for your safe little bubble. Don't drink alcohol? Then drop something else, such as coffee. The key is to test your self control.
- **Do the unwanted task –** Those situations always arise when something not ideal or easy has to be done yet everyone avoids doing it. Be the person to step forward and do it, every time. For example, remember as a kid when the ball would go over the fence to the grumpy neighbour's backyard and everyone was too scared to get it? Be that guy with the balls to do it.
- **Genuinely ask a stranger or homeless person how they are –** Most people are too wrapped up in their own lives to talk to strangers let alone homeless dudes. It's uncomfortable too. Take 5 minutes and have a *real* conversation.
- **Single men: approach 5 strangers this week and practice your game –** Not only will it push the comfort zone, but it will infinitely help you improve your game. No outcome *intended* other than a chat.
- **Taken men: approach 5 people that could help you in some way –** This could be with anything, such as a business partnership or an acquaintance that you know is great with kids so you and the other half can enjoy some quality child free time. Get outside your comfort zone and start making shit happen.
- **Set up a meeting with someone that can advance**

your career or business – Too many people roll along accepting the status quo and waiting for others to *give* them opportunities. We all make our own fate, go and make some opportunities happen. Hustle. As Daniel Priestly, author of *Entrepreneur Revolution* says, "Make your own luck".

• **Jump out of a plane –** self-explanatory.

"You'll miss the best things if you keep your eyes shut."

– DR. SEUSS

Plan and go on holidays – Your time on this earth is about living a wonderful *life*, not necessarily just a wonderful retirement. So make sure you go on holidays every year and spend some concentrated time chilling out, on adventures, whatever floats your boat. *"All work and no play makes* (insert your name here) *a dull boy"* remember.

Make a list of the things you love most – This can be people, activities, whatever. List them and start prioritising them in your life and getting them into your week.

Act like a child from time to time – Most of us have serious lives with serious jobs where we have to be serious to other serious people. Acting like an immature child every now and then is a vital way to stay young and keep your mind light and joyful. I consider myself to be professional and carry myself in a manner that sets examples for my clients and readers, however, I *still* laugh and act like a ridiculous idiot often. Don't be afraid to be immature sometimes.

Daily enjoyment diary – You should be filling this out by now, but ensure you keep a detailed account of what you enjoy each day and the things you wish you could be doing. And... *do them!*

To discover your inner Alpha you must prioritise enjoyment, fun, and love in your life. If something gives you the shits and is causing constant stress then it's going to fight against anything else you may be doing in your life to improve yourself. Start getting comfortable, being uncomfortable. You'll soon see yourself change and grow with your inner Alpha shining through. You'll start enjoying life and all sorts of awesome stuff will be happening.

***

Here's a philosophy to adopt – Ensure that you get enough quality sleep, have a positive attitude and outlook on life, try to do things you enjoy every day, don't sweat the small stuff, prioritise your health, enjoyment and spending time with family, loved ones, and friends. Always try to put time into yourself and make sure you're doing what makes *you* happy and prioritise yourself. Strive to do great things for others, but never neglect yourself.

Always look after number one!

"Believe me! The secret of reaping the greatest fruitfulness and the greatest enjoyment from life is to live dangerously!"
– FRIEDRICH NIETZSCHE

MAN SKILLS

OPERATING LIKE A GENTLEMAN – BECOMING A LEGEND

"People are often unreasonable and self-centred. Forgive them anyway. If you are kind, people may accuse you of ulterior motives. Be kind anyway. If you are honest, people may cheat you. Be honest anyway. If you find happiness, people may be jealous. Be happy anyway. The good you do today may be forgotten tomorrow. Do good anyway. Give the world the best you have, and it may never be enough. Give your best anyway"

– MOTHER TERESA

Can we tell the essence of a man from what he eats or how he trains? Can we *really* know what he's like by how much quality sleep he gets or his personal goals? **No.**

These are definitely crucial factors in shaping and moulding a man. Without these we can't become a real Alpha, *our Alpha*. However, for you to truly discover and unleash your inner Alpha, you must have the finer points of manhood down. These details have to be part of your repertoire, entrenched in your psyche and in a holster so efficient that once in a fitted tuxedo you could be mistaken for (a less 1960's) James Bond.

Ask anyone who is attracted to men what it is, besides abs, "guns" and a great smile, that attracts and hooks them to a guy. *Personality*, or a combination of terms that fall into this umbrella is what will ring true.

This doesn't just mean the ability to make a girl laugh or entertain a crowd. This means a man's beliefs, his virtues and the way he acts and carries himself on a daily basis. Not only when around people, but even when no one's watching.

We touched on the definition of our Alpha at the start of this book – *a man knows who he is, knows how to deal with his emotions, face his fears and can stand resolute when needed, hold his own in conversation and do so with compassion, integrity and humility.*

This man is a leader. He's courageous, has his shit sorted and has strength of character, mind, and body. He is confident, self-assured, and willing to step into the unknown. This is a man with appeal, a man who knows himself, knows how he operates best and knows what he's doing in this world. This is a man who knows his A-game and uses it to benefit himself *and* others every day. This is a man with game, appeal, control, and conviction. This is *our Alpha.*

So, once you've got your head right, started eating how a man should, training like a beast and sorted out your sleep and stress to become a much happier dude, how do you refine and ensure you can tick off the Alpha criteria?

This can be a tricky one, as it's usually something that comes from our upbringing. However, you must embrace change to grow and improve. *We* choose our fate and life, so developing some of these skills and traits that may be lacking can be done. Like anything else we've seen, it doesn't have to be complicated, but it may require some hard work!

PERSONAL BRAND AND THE FINER POINTS OF BEING A MAN

"Clothes make the man. Naked people have little or no influence on society."

– MARK TWAIN

To master your domain, fine tune your game, and become a man people just want to be around, you must first realise that you are a brand. To be more precise, *you are your own brand.* Everything that you do, say, and act out is living 3D advertising of your brand as a man.

This is what dictates how people interact with you and how they piece together your personality and behavioural traits, whether consciously or not. People form opinions of others literally within seconds, so the image that fronts you *must* be on the money.

Unless you're consciously aware of this yourself and act to a certain brand all the time, you need to start making some changes to chisel, sculpt, and improve the image you're putting out to the world with your every breath.

As much as you can control your own fate, you're still what others say about you.

This concept of reputation is one held in the highest of regard by some and given little or no weight by others. For budding Alphas it needs to be at the forefront of almost everything you do. Without a rock solid and awesome reputation you'll never master your own game and create a personal brand that has you kicking goals in all areas of your life. The two go hand in hand.

The first thing to master when it comes to your man brand is to **always be at your authentic best.** This can be a tricky one and will undoubtedly have its less than ideal moments, but if you attack each day with the motto of *always being at your authentic best* then you will actively pursue that and it will start to be present in all of your actions.

There are endless examples of how this applies, like dealing with your boss, approaching a potential partner, or simply hanging out with your mates. Either way, being at your best will become what others think about you and in turn what they say about you. Therefore strengthening your reputation and personal brand. This also means being authentic – not lying or pretending to be something you're not.

This goes for how you act towards and deal with others as well as yourself. We've covered being the best for you with your daily mindset, nutrition, training, sleep and enjoying life, now it requires being your best in the other areas of your life *and* towards others, improving your emotional intelligence.

In order for you to be able to give your best to others you must first give the best to yourself. This means *being selfish!* Always look after number one. If you don't put concerted effort into yourself then you'll never be at your best. If you're not at your best then you can't do your best, to, and for others, you're short changing the world of the full you.

Schedule time each day purely for yourself and be ruthless with it. Remove distractions and put some work into yourself. This may be as simple as scheduling regular workouts, sleep, reading, or meal times for some. For others it might mean sitting in a quiet spot and just chilling out and "being present", rather than *doing*.

Having regular alone time is missing these days, so make sure you chill by yourself with just your thoughts and do it regularly. Put great importance on this stuff and don't let anything short of an emergency change it.

This also goes for doing stuff you don't want to do or that is going to mess up your "me time." To ensure this, next time you get invited to something you'd rather not attend and that's encroaching on me time, just say "no thanks."

Being selfish in this way doesn't have to be acting like an arsehole, nor is it an excuse to be one. You are doing this to prioritise yourself when it's scheduled and needed. You still have to help out and chip in and act with empathy.

Acting with honesty and integrity are crucial factors in any Alpha. Honesty being the best policy doesn't always hold true, of course we know that at times we must bend the truth slightly to protect others.

However, outside of those moments you must strive to use honesty wherever possible. Little white lies sneak into our days all the time and it's usually to spare others or ourselves some level of pain. What we're really doing is holding back our true opinion while demeaning our relationships and interactions. Try to tell the truth where possible. It may be uncomfortable at times but it will result in better connections with people and you'll find it very liberating not holding in key thoughts and emotions.

Further from this is **acting with integrity and authenticity and being a man of your word.** There are many terrible things in this world, but when it comes to day-to-day interacting with others, few are worse than being let down by someone on their promise. This also goes for your day-to-day interactions with people, be it colleagues, employees, loved ones or strangers. Always strive to act with integrity and authenticity.

To develop a strong personal brand and a reputation that has others talking about you in a way that has people gravitating towards you, you must act with care, kindness, compassion, and integrity. The best lesson I ever learnt from my amazing mother was that **manners cost you nothing, but get you the world.** This is something that has been lost on current generations as countless children and adolescents push their way through crowded streets and walk through doorways held open for them without a simple acknowledgement or thank you.

Using great manners when dealing with someone you've met will give a great first impression, just as using them with a close friend will strengthen their opinion and view of you. This is an integral part of who you are as a man and therefore the brand that you put out to the world. This goes for acting like an old school gentleman as well – something that isn't always necessary, but can add the spark to a moment that would be bland without it.

Remember that going the extra mile or doing the unexpected is what makes you stand out from the crowd and gives you added appeal.

This also goes for complimenting people. Some find receiving compliments awkward, however, that doesn't mean they don't like getting them. It feels awesome to get great feedback from people, so start doing it for others. Just make sure it's genuine.

Seems simple, but this is the kind of behaviour that is missing from today's anti-Alpha, especially on a consistent and long-term basis. Remember that vulnerability is strength, so start practising it.

"Tenderness and kindness are not signs of weakness and despair but manifestations of strength and resolution."

– KAHLIL GIBRAN

Just as being gracious, kind, and caring is important to our Alpha, so is knowing when to take a stand and stick up for what you believe in. Having backbone and spirit is crucial to discovering and producing your inner Alpha on a regular basis. This doesn't mean be a stubborn arsehole that never backs down; it means knowing when to choose your battles and then how to play it out.

If you make a stand, then make sure you do just that. If you're to win an argument that needs winning or stick up for your rights or those of others in need, do so with energy and intensity.

It's best not to have enemies, but if someone crosses you in a manner that requires you to fight, take it to them, but do it with honour and integrity. If you win, move on, be humble and don't rub it in. If you lose, or it turns out that you were wrong; admit it, apologise if necessary and be a gracious loser. People will take note when you fight for what you believe in, so the manner in which you go about this will be watched and either admired or loathed.

Always be on time wherever possible. Some people don't value this very highly, and that's fine if it's something that only involves them. But if any occasion involves one or more other people then there's a very good chance that some or all of them *will* value punctuality and not being kept waiting.

Therefore, you should strive to be on time for every interaction with another human being. This doesn't mean you have to be early, it just means be on time and don't keep people waiting. In doing this you're being respectful of the person you're connecting with and being respectful of your own brand.

Being known as the person that's always late does nothing to strengthen your personal brand. If you're late for whatever reason, take responsibility for it – don't blame the traffic or whatever else. Own it.

Regardless of your religious or spiritual beliefs, acting with kindness to anyone you meet or deal with will come back around to you in some way, shape, or form. **At the very least it will strengthen your brand and reputation.** Be nice to strangers as well as the people closest to you. Perform random acts of kindness on a daily basis.

> *"It's not what you do when people are watching, it's what you do when you're alone that defines the person you are or will become."*
>
> – UNKNOWN TO THE AUTHOR

How you act is vital to the perception others have about you. However, after that you must present a great brand, one that's appealing to the eye as well as the mind and heart. We've covered how to get in great shape, how to feel amazing, and how to have awesome energy all day every day, but there's more to it than just looking good naked. Although this does rate highly on most people's radar and definitely for any aspiring Alphas!

You must also know how to present yourself in the best light possible when it comes to your brand. So when you go to work, don't just look the part, *look sharp*. When you head out with a girl, don't just look good, look awesome. When you go for a coffee, make sure if you run into a potential client, they will definitely want to work with you.

Looking the part is a crucial part of your brand and reputation. This isn't to say you must have the reputation of someone who is a style innovator, fashion leader, or conceited, simply that you look good and take great care of yourself.

What we're talking about here is personal grooming, appropriate dress sense, and overall style. As to present a great visual brand you must get to know your body and what works with it and how you look best. If you're as gifted in the height department as Tom Cruise then avoid wearing long shirts un-tucked – it will make you look shorter. If you've got the "bean pole" stature of a marathon runner then wearing a suit that isn't fitted will make you look like a 10 year-old who's dressed up in dad's clothes.

There are endless examples of what *not* to do, but you have to know your body and learn what will suit it best. This can be the difference between looking good and looking so damn good that people are approaching you at random.

We'll cover over some of the keys below, however, if you go to your bonus material you'll find much more in-depth information on all of this personal style stuff, such as grooming, facial hair, and dress. Sounds like "goes without saying" kind of stuff, but sadly so many guys let themselves down here. *Don't be that guy.*

We've covered a few topics in this brand and reputation section, so let's look at your key points and strategies as well as the key personal style take homes.

PERSONAL BRAND AND REPUTATION STRATEGIES

1. Always be at your best
2. Always look after number one
3. Honesty and integrity rule

4. Manners cost you nothing, but get you the world
5. If something requires a fight then give it your best, but be gracious and civil
6. Always be on time
7. Treat others as you want to be treated
8. Go the extra mile and do the unexpected
9. Clothes make the man – There's a reason this saying dates back to the middle-ages, because people judge a book by its cover, or in our case a man by his clothes. Always dress for the occasion and never be under-dressed. Make sure you work out your body shape and dress to enhance it, not hide it. Specifics are in your bonus material.
10. Style your hair to suit *you* not the trends
11. Basic grooming is a must
12. Have a cologne that attracts people to you

These are some baseline keys for personal brand, grooming and presenting an appealing man to the world. This is your brand – your man brand. Make sure you look good and present a gentleman and a legend.

"There is nothing noble in being superior to your fellow man; true nobility is being superior to your former self."

– ERNEST HEMMINGWAY

***

To become a true Alpha you must create an awesome brand out of yourself and you must work at it. Things like this don't just happen for a lot of us (unless you're Johnny Depp) and we have to work at it. Starting each day with a positive and happy frame of mind with the intent to do great things will go a long way towards kicking that off. Just make sure that your intention is to be the best version of *you*, not someone else. Comparing yourself to others is a futile pursuit that will only lead to dissatisfaction. Be the best *you*.

For you to get up to scratch with your personal brand and implement some of these key strategies to increase and improve your reputation and become a legend, there are some challenges for you to start completing. Turn to the back of this chapter to see your '*Man Skills challenges*'.

Every man should aim to leave this world better than when he entered it. Your actions and the way you treat people will determine this.

> *"When we look at modern man, we have to face the fact that modern man suffers from a kind of poverty of the spirit, which stand in glaring contrast with a scientific and technological abundance. We've learned to fly the air as birds, we've learned to swim the seas as fish, yet we haven't learned to walk the Earth as brothers and sisters."*
>
> – MARTIN LUTHER KING JR

DEVELOPING STRONG BONDS AND RELATIONSHIPS

"You are the average of the five people you spend the most time with."

– JIM ROHN

To kick it off we'll look at how to approach things in a romantic relationship. As elements of this are going to be key for any single man wanting to land himself a partner, be it long term or very short. Just as they are for your dealings with a current partner and anyone else close to you, such as a parent, a sibling, a child, a mate, or a colleague.

We'll talk about this in relation to females. However, as we saw much earlier on this information applies to both straight and gay men, as we're essentially talking about masculine and feminine energies. It would be remiss of me to start dishing out specific advice to gay men about dealing with other gay men. In that, I am not practised. So from now on if it applies to you read "female," "women," "her," etc, as the *feminine*.

One thing many men do when they're in a relationship is hold back. They're tentative and withdrawn and the other person never really knows how they feel. This is understandable from a point of view that you may not be too sure exactly how you feel about them. However, to have successful relationships we must start to evaluate these connections and decide whether we want them to continue, because if not and they proceed, people will get hurt.

The simple way to figure this out is have some alone time, think about what you want out of a relationship with a certain person, how you feel about them, and how they make you feel. If the answers are all positive then you need to proceed with positive action.

This doesn't mean being over the top, clingy and needy. That shit's not cool. It just means embracing vulnerability and *letting that person know how you feel.*

Of course if this person is someone you're already in an established relationship with then you definitely need to let them know, regularly, that you care about them and they are important to you.

Think about it from your own perspective – do you like to be told or shown that you're special by someone? Then chances are the other person does too. Leaving them to guess is a losing strategy.

This is where individual love languages come in. In his book, *The 5 Love Languages,* Gary Chapman explains that the different languages people use to show love and appreciation and how reading other people's signs is our preferred subconscious way of receiving affection. This provides great insight into how you show love (and affection) and like to receive it from others, as well as how others express their own feelings.

The 5 languages are:

- **Words of affirmation –** this language uses words to affirm people
- **Quality time –** this language is all about giving the

person your undivided attention
- **Receiving gifts –** for some people what makes them feel most loved is to receive a gift
- **Acts of service –** for these people actions speak louder than words
- **Physical touch –** to this person nothing speaks more deeply than appropriate touch

To have truly happy, awesome, and powerful relationships both sexual and not, you must know how best to act towards an individual and what makes them tick. It's no use trying to stubbornly make them fit to your way of seeing things. For example, if they predominantly resonate with small regular gifts but you like to share how important they are to you with words, all the dialogue from you to them won't cut it. They need small gifts to show appreciation while you need to be affirmed with words.

Regardless of someone's natural method of expressing love, care, affection and respect, you must endeavour to express that to them, ideally in a manner that resonates with them.

This will encourage, foster and build strong relationships. This will strengthen your connections and they'll have a natural reaction that, "this person really gets me."

A true Alpha who has his A-game down knows how to talk to and act around people in a manner that shows care, understanding and empathy. This results in people being drawn to you and wanting to interact with you. This is the game of *Our Alpha*.

One important thing to note when it comes to relationships of love is that a great connection and having a strong bond with someone should be a prerequisite for a solid and happy union. You should enjoy spending time with your partner, *and want to.*

So many guys find setting aside time for "the Mrs" to be a massive drag. *Why on earth are you with them in the first place?* You should *want* to hang out with them and have fun with them – travel, holiday, party, and chill with them. If this is a pain in the arse, then question why you're with them at all because it's going to be hard being happy long term without these elements.

This is where the idea of your partner being your best friend comes in. Of course, if you're in a relationship for a bit of fun and it's mutually accepted as being that much, then cool, there's no need for this. However, if you're with someone long term, or plan on it being that way, they should be your best friend.

The key point here is that *she's your best friend*, **not your mate.**

Your mates are the boys; we all know what "the boys" entails. It's different for some guys that may not have many male friends, but the way a group of guy mates act towards each other is different to how you should act towards your partner. So don't treat her as a mate, playing pranks on her that will actually embarrass her or cause emotional pain.

The boys can handle this stuff. Your lady friend should be absent from this, otherwise it leads to the relationship becoming easy and taken for granted. This will cause any spark to be lost and soon you're in a stale relationship with little or no chemistry from where things only go downhill badly.

Make sure your partner is your best friend, but don't treat her like the boys.

Of special note here is that this isn't all about touching base with your feminine, we want balance remember. So having your "man time" with the boys is a crucial part of that. It allows the pure masculine to come out. Your mates will keep you in check and provide an outlet for the kind of behaviour your partner should be exempt from.

***

In much the same way, knowing your partner's love language will help to enhance and strengthen any current or forming romantic and sexual relationships. It will also help the single man when he deals with potential partners. If you can recognise someone's dominant language and act accordingly they will feel your understanding of them and be more open and trusting.

Be it conscious or not, women have a check list in their brain when it comes to choosing a mate and the more you can score points on that board, the more she'll let you in and the better connection you'll have. Ergo, good things happen.

One of the key elements to winning over a potential partner or ensuring continual respect from a current one is to have confidence. Talk to any female and ask her to rank her top 3 traits in a guy. Confidence will come up more often than not. However, this is something that many guys lack and struggle to grasp the concept of.

For us, *this is one of the main traits needed to truly reach the point of knowing your inner Alpha.* Confidence can be present in many different ways, depending on the man and the situation, the main thing to note is that you must have it!

Confidence, without arrogance is an Alpha must have <== tweet that shit! @mcampbell2012 #UnleashYourAlpha

If you're in a relationship and you lack confidence then it's safe to say you don't wear the pants, and I bet it gets to you from time to time; maybe a lot of the time.

Maybe you've never thought about it. If not, do so now. The only way to claw your way back and gain some control and respect is to start acting with confidence. There should be an equal proportion of pant wearing, but for the most part as a strong Alpha, you should be able to take control of situations and simply *be the man*.

Women want this but generally don't get it and have had to play that masculine part, hence them wearing the pants. Women will respect a man who stands up for what he believes, acts with integrity, conviction and can take charge. To do this you must have confidence. This isn't overt arrogance, but a subtle confidence that says:

'Don't worry, I've got this shit' **<=== add this to your vocab immediately!**

This is your masculine coming to the fore.

In just the same way as a married man may need to step up and win the respect of his wife by discovering his confidence and *mojo*, so too does the single man looking to pick up. This isn't just how you talk or behave in social situations, but how you hold yourself. This goes for all budding Alphas – posture and how you hold your physical self is the start of exuding self-assuredness. From here your actions and words will back that up.

So if you're a guy that struggles to talk to women unless you've smashed ten beers already, then you need to start getting *way* outside your comfort zone and thus, using your balls! You need to start putting yourself into the kind of situations where you can talk to women sober. Not only will you grow as a person, but you'll also talk to more women and usually hit a better quality of interaction than a drunken and possibly regrettable hook-up.

It will be hard and you'll get rejected, no doubt, but without going through that process you'll never develop the confidence required to do it effectively and more effortlessly.

(Read more on this from Mike here: **unleashyouralpha.com/ i'm-just-not-that-confident-with-chicks)*

That's what we all want isn't it? To be able to stroll confidently into a room, see a smoking hot woman and approach her? That's balls and that is how a real Alpha goes about getting the things he wants – with conviction and *cajones!* It's not necessary of course, but if it's doable you should be able to do it. It's very much part of the Alpha journey.

The question at this point is usually – **how do you get confidence like that if the mere idea scares you?**

This may be very individual, however, there are a few key things to realise and from there it's simply a process of application.

The keys to gaining confidence with women (and life):

Women are friendly, social creatures that want to talk to people and interact just like you want to with them. This means that if you're out somewhere and you see a girl you'd like to talk to, the chances are that she'd like to have a chat with someone too. *So go do it.* Realising that chicks are open to chat, especially to great guys who have their shit sorted (that's you) breaks down the imaginary wall many guys think exist. **Take home: women generally want to meet great guys as much as we want to meet great chicks, so start approaching them AND SMILE!**

You will get rejected, but that's okay. No one can be liked by absolutely everyone, that includes you, and nor should you want to. Rejection is a form of failure and failure is how we learn and grow. If you try talking to one girl and it doesn't go well, this shouldn't be a reason to get down or embarrassed, you need to learn from the situation and move on to the next. **Take home: rejection should provide lessons so you can improve and grow for next time.**

Only asking questions that you're sure of hearing a yes to will limit your experiences. Fearing hearing the word *no* stops us from acting. However, once you realise that to hear no is fine, you'll be clear of this often paralysing fear and have the balls to start asking more questions. Without asking the question you're never any better off. **Take home: if you never ask, then you'll never know.**

Nothing great ever happens inside your comfort zone. To achieve great things you have to stretch yourself and this means getting outside your comfort zone. You may never get comfortable approaching girls sober or off the cuff, but that doesn't mean you shouldn't take a leap and do it.

Once you realise that awesome things can happen when you're nervous or pushed to your limits and that you will feel this way when you do uncomfortable things; like approaching a girl in the supermarket, or telling your partner what you really want sexually, you'll know that the feeling you have is all part of it. **Take home: getting outside your comfort zone with things like talking to women may always be nerve racking, but it's exhilarating and an awesome way to grow confidence as a man. No one will help you, you just have to man up and do it.**

Conquering the things you fear the most will unlock your inner confidence. If you have a fear of something then attacking it head on will open your eyes to a confidence you may not have known you had. Scared of sharks? Go for an ocean swim at night. The adrenaline alone will carry you through and you'll soon find something like chatting to your crush to be a walk in the park. **Take home: developing balls in one area will carry over to confidence in others.**

Posture and holding yourself in a confident manner does half the job. Recent studies have shown that holding a strong and confident posture works to increase your testosterone. This automatically makes you more appealing to the opposite sex (or whoever you're looking to attract) as well as presenting a strong and desirable potential partner or mate. **Take home: to get eyes on you, you must hold yourself with confidence and this includes good posture.**

Worrying about your looks or whether you're good enough has lost you the race already. If you think you're not good enough for someone then you're not. You must believe in yourself, your looks, your personality, your brand, and your game. This will exude a subtle confidence and someone who is happy in their skin. If you worry that you don't look good enough or have great chat then potential mates will easily pick this up. **Take home: have faith in the work you're doing elsewhere that the hard work shows. You're looking good and you're a great catch.**

Listen more than you talk. This doesn't mean you can't talk at all; you should simply be attentive, ask about her and let the conversation flow from her answers. Keep chat about yourself to a minimum. Ask more open-ended questions than you answer. **Take home: most people like to talk about themselves, so ask about her and *listen intently.***

Be interesting. There's nothing worse than a guy who makes crappy, boring small talk, or tries the same old pick up lines. Stand out from the crowd and be memorable. If this doesn't come naturally, then plan some conversation starters, such as "Where is the one place on earth you would *least* like to travel?", or, "Given an unlimited budget, what would you do tomorrow?"

Once you start to make these realisations, you must then apply the principles of them. This means not fearing rejection and just walking into a room with your head high and prepared to walk up to a girl and start a conversation. Feel free to have a conversation starter ready to go after a friendly greeting, but don't try too hard. A chick isn't looking for an instant comedian – yeah it may help, but just being genuine and listening with intent will get you into many a friendly situation and on the front foot. If not, learn from it and move on.

On the subject of conversation starters, this is something crucial to master. I've included a specific technique in your bonus *Man Skills* material.

Confidence is *the absolute key* to getting anywhere. Women sense it and it fuels you to do things you may never have dreamed of in the past. Confidence and masculine appeal are a huge factor in women choosing a mate, be it long term or very short.

***

Having great connections with women isn't just about talking or acting in the right way in certain situations, it's also about having awesome, out of this world *sex*. What we learn in porn films as young walking erections is that women are to be aggressively dominated for our pleasure first and foremost. *This is absolute bollocks!*

In case you hadn't realised, porn isn't a real life sexual instructional video. For the most part the way to a women's sexual heart is through a deep emotional connection, trust, and setting an environment that allows her to relax and completely let go.

Creating passion in bed will translate directly to happiness in your relationship and it's noticeable to the contrary. If a woman is unsatisfied sexually then it will be evident in the day to day of your life. She'll make you pay for it, emotionally. *Who wants that?*

Women can be complicated and confusing, however, if you treat her right, she'll be a loyal and trusting partner. On the other hand, if she is neglected life can become unhappy for all involved. To satisfy her and meet her needs, you must treat her her right; that means security, great chemistry and at times awesome, neighbour-disturbing sex.

That may mean deep, silky love making, but it also means raw, emotional, passionate, sweaty and wild sexual adventure; one she'll remember forever. Routine and end-result focus are a sure-fire way to lose passion and connection and create a very frustrated, unsatisfied, and irritable person.

For women, sexual gratification can come in many forms, and the simple act itself will usually garner a decent level of pleasure. However, for a woman to have a mind-blowing orgasm, one that will literally make her weak at the knees (and a huge fan of yours), she must be able to *let go*.

She has to be able to trust you enough to be completely vulnerable and free of emotional barriers. This will lead to incredible sex and your assertion as a true Alpha in her life. She won't feel the remotest need to even look for anyone else; when she's comfortable with you she's more likely to invest further in your connection.

This comes down to your physical appearance, confidence, behaviours, social status, and reputation. If she knows you're someone people like being around and want to deal with, someone who has passion, loves what he does, and does great things, then she'll be more impressed and feel special because you've chosen her. That might sound a bit sexist or derogatory, but it's not. It's a primal human behaviour. Put yourself in those shoes and it works too. The animal world is consistent with choosing mates throughout time.

For the most part this comes down to all the behavioural aspects we've covered already, however, there are obvious and decisive factors that come into play once the clothes come off and the wheels of bodily fluid take motion.

Without making this a complete "how-to guide" and getting into sweaty and sticky detail, let's cover some key fundamentals to make you a better lover and make her (or him) want you all the more:

Connect – This is the start of the experience. Of course fast, spontaneous, and furious is sometimes best, but if you think of the most powerful experiences you've had, chances are planning was involved. This is crucial for women – she needs to be able to relax, be comfortable and to make an emotional connection with you. If she's still got the day's worries on her mind, nothing will get her to ecstasy. However coming home to a clean house with scented candles lit, a glass of her favourite wine and a head massage (or preference) will help to light the embers she needs to be able to let go and be in the moment.

Foreplay first – Unlike us, women usually need some warming up – time to get the mind in the game and the emotions tied into the act. Obviously, her body reacts on a physiological level in this way too, and needs some "greasing of the wheels" so to speak. Not every time of course, but consider that she needs more time than you to get fully turned on and ready for the main act.

Take your time and get her both physically and mentally ready. Once you've set the scene and made a connection, slowly touch her everywhere, brush past her most sensitive spots, but don't just establish a new permanent base there. She should be close to, if not audibly begging you to fuck her. Make sure you listen to your gut with this; don't second-guess yourself.

Take charge – Of course there's no absolutes with anything, especially sex, but women want a man that can take charge in the bedroom, control the proceedings, and let them relax and enjoy it. This won't be the case all the time but you have to be able to throw her down on the bed, rip her clothes off and get animalistic. It's hot and she'll be putty in your hands.

Be a selfless lover – Again, this won't be all the time but if you set out with her interests at heart yours will be well and truly taken care of. Your aim should be to get her off, or at least show her a *very* good time. This also goes for timing – she may be up for it and you're not really. In this case always remember that when you're as randy as a teenage rabbit and she's not quite in the mood, she probably does her part to satisfy you. Find the time *she* loves to have sex and make it happen.

The clitoris is queen – Every man should have this location etched in their subconscious, especially for their partner's needs. This requires attention and the right kind. Pressure, speed, and motion are key.

Communicate – Don't quite know how she likes to be touched or licked? Then ask. Every woman is different, and no "standard move" will work on everyone, so you must learn to be open and communicate with a partner to find out exactly what it is that sends them screaming the roof off. Just as you should be able to express what you like and what she can do to make things better for you.

Love to have sex – This seems almost backwards right? But there's a huge difference between getting yourself off and having an awesome sexual experience with a partner.

Getting a chick naked and stumbling through a sexual encounter is a sure fire way to turn her off. To have real game and create excellent relationships, you need to take control and ensure any sexual event has her coming back for more and singing your praises to her friends (because she will). Work on these essentials and start finding your sexual game too; your confidence and personal brand will flourish.

***

We've seen how reading someone's love language will strengthen your bond with them. The same applies for any kind of business, client, or professional relationship as well as dealing with your mates or a blossoming bromance. Yep, bromances are real and need just the same kind of care and attention as a romance (except for the sex).

These languages carry over to all relationships with the obvious difference being the type of connection. So, if you're dealing with your boss and can't seem to make sense of their behaviour towards you, or you can't seem to get your professional feelings across, then the same kind of behaviours and reactions from the love languages are relevant.

You might be telling a client how much you appreciate them by saying it and sharing it with others, but if this isn't their "appreciation language" then it'll fall on deaf ears. They might value quality time, so that's what they need from you to see how much you appreciate their business: time.

Think of any situations where you've done something for a mate and they haven't reacted. They *might* be emotionally inept, but also your act, words or whatever, may have been missed because they don't operate in that space. So, buying him a box of beers for helping you move might not cut it because he reacts to physical touch. He just needed a heartfelt hug, some genuine man love. Nothing wrong with that!

The next level here for any budding Alpha is to understand bromances and how to go about them. This might be as simple as dealing with a current mate, but a budding bromance is a new man-to-man friendship in the making. For this to form and the *bromance* to become official – a close relationship between two bros is established to such a point where the bros seem like a couple. If this is a relationship that you want to form, then you need to treat it like trying to win over a chick.

If you're attempting to win the affection of a girl then don't go head first in and be super keen or ask for the goods straight away. This will usually raise alarms and send her running for the metaphorical hills. You must do the same for a budding bromance. Flirting in a bromance kind of way is needed, as well as not acting too keen or too comfortable early on.

To establish a bromance with a guy you'd like to become mates with or simply develop some kind of professional relationship with, then you have to follow the same steps you would with a female and use your A-game. So, go back to the steps laid out on the previous pages; use your challenges (coming up), knowledge of the different appreciation languages, and be a great guy. Failing at nailing a bromance is failing with your game.

You need to start treating the relationships in your life; from a girl you'd like to connect with sexually, to a potential client, with the same kind of attention, care, understanding, and behaviour. All of this will build consistency in your personal brand, which will in turn strengthen your reputation while cementing some quality relationships in your life. This is how our Alpha behaves and operates – *like a gentleman.*

This stuff can be a bit confusing and overwhelming if you try to analyse every person you deal with. However, the best steps forward here are baby ones. Nail a few key elements and move on to new ones.

Keep notes and refer to them in time to see where you've come from and how things have changed. This will also serve to show you your strengths and weaknesses and therefore, the areas that need the most work.

MAN SKILLS CHALLENGES: PART 1

Qualities of a real Alpha – Go back to the activity from the start of this book where you wrote down what you thought it meant to be a man and what you perceived your own characteristics to be. Now. Now do this again, but also write down what you think you need to improve. Have a look at how these compare to the description of our Alpha and your own.

Write out a 'Rules to live by' – This isn't mine or someone else's, these are *your* rules to live by. Rules, thoughts, and guidelines that govern your everyday decisions. They may be things that apply now or have applied in the past. They may also be things you wish to start doing or behaviours you'd like to emulate. Either way, make a list and aim for at least 50. This can be extremely powerful and enlightening. *Remember*, you have to follow them. I've included my current rules in the bonus material for reference.

*(Also see Mike's Rule's To Live By here: **unleashyouralpha.com/ what-would-mike-do**)*

Do something nice for a stranger once a day – This can be as small as giving some food to a homeless guy or helping an old lady with her groceries, to helping out at a shelter or paying for a student's petrol.

Do something nice anonymously for someone you know daily – This means that you don't tell them or brag about it, just do it because it's a good thing to do.

Give 5 compliments daily – These must be truthful and genuine. Try making someone's day, watch their face light up and see how you feel after that. Brightening someone's day is a sure fire way to brighten your own.

The purely positive day – This means that for an entire day you speak and think nothing but positives – no criticisms, no complaining, no whining, no insults, no snarky comments, no self-loathing. Sticking with only positive chat will help shift your frame of mind and make you realise that most things we bitch about are pointless, petty energy suckers.

Choose 5 people from different areas in your life to learn their language – A romantic interest or partner, a friend, a family member, a colleague, and someone who you'd like to get closer to. Start looking at your interactions and take a mental note of how they react to your behaviour towards them. Once you can nail down their language and subsequently act in ways that enhance that, they will consciously or subconsciously know that you "get them." This makes for great relationships and real A-game.

Attend a networking event, be it personal or business – Networking events can be an awesome way to talk to a whole bunch of strangers in a short time. It forces you to make conversation, talk to strangers, and aids in growing your confidence. If you're a single man go to some speed dating nights (*sober*) and literally practise your game. The forced interaction and quick turnover is awesome for building confidence talking to women. If you're attached, then go to some networking events. Have a think about what you're going to talk about, but this should be personal brand marketing.

Get rejected – Purposely go out to a social setting with the plan of getting rejected. Be a bit over the top and ballsy. Really listen to what the other person says and learn from it. Regardless of whether you act like your normal self or not, what they say will give you vital information about how to act in the future.

Ask 3 people what they *really* think of you – Choose three people from different areas of your life - home, work, social - and ask them to go away and think about what they truthfully think of you, both pros and cons. You are to listen to the feedback and take it on board. No excuses or getting defensive; just listen and take note. This will give you some valuable insight into what the world thinks your personal brand is.

Improve personal brand – For your confidence to grow and your behaviour as a real Alpha to flourish, you *must* work on your personal brand. If that means getting in shape, then get cracking although you should be onto that already! If it means changing what people say about you, then pull your head in and start acting in a way that will achieve positive change.

Conquer another fear – As mentioned above, to gain confidence with the ladies, think of something that scares the crap out of you and go and do it. Then keep doing it and other things – this attitude will carry over to all aspects of your life.

Sex – If you're single this might be harder, excuse the pun, than for the attached men, but to gain true inner Alpha confidence and get the woman (or man) in your life shouting your praises from the rooftops, then you need to master the "sexy time." The key to this is asking questions, listening intently and putting the lessons into practice. Whatever they're after, as long as it's legal, then start doing it.

Five Questions – The conversation starter. Check your bonus material for this.

And that is our definitive guide to getting the confidence of a real Alpha, learning how to read lovers and the people in your life and fine tuning your A-game to kick goals elsewhere in your life.

"In every industry, there is an edge. In your business or personal life it doesn't matter – somewhere there is a cliff. Most people don't want to be close to it, because they're afraid they'll fall off.
Thing is, the edge is where all the cool stuff happens."

- JULIEN SMITH

"Success is not a result of spontaneous combustion. You must set yourself on fire."

- REGGIE LEACH

YOUR INNER 007

*"...when men are growing up and are reading about Batman, Spiderman, Superman...these aren't fantasies. **These are options.** This is the deep inner secret truth of the male mind."*

– JERRY SEINFELD

When we're born, it's obvious that we have the parts that label us male. The things between our legs ensure that we fall into the hairier half of our species.

From this moment we grow, develop and become boys. Depending on each situation, we start to take on some traits, characteristics, and behaviours of grown men.

As we've seen already, today's boys are arguably lacking real and appropriate role models and are often influenced heavily or disproportionately by the women and anti-Alphas in their lives. We're hitting the point at which we see one bearing the age of a man but perhaps not the status of a man and this is where some of the finer points come in to play that make up "man cred."

When you grew up did you learn how to back a trailer? How to bait a hook? Or even how to cook a steak properly? These are the kind of things we pick up as we grow through boyhood into adolescence and then manhood. They are the extra little skills and talents that every man should "just know."

So, regardless of what your upbringing was, if you went on to become a mechanic, a lawyer or a chef we're looking to develop you into a well-rounded guy, one that has the confidence in any situation he finds himself in. Your day job may mean that you can change a tire with your eyes closed, put on a 5 star feed or negotiate the sale of goose down jackets to African tribesman, but if you don't have an array of various skills up your sleeve that mark you as a man then your Alpha pedigree isn't complete. Some of these are a bit of fun, but these are your shoeshine, your topcoat, and your finishing school.

What we're going to look at in this section is exactly that, those skills that make us men and ensure that, you too, have an appropriate level of *James Bond* and *Batman* in you.

Over the next few pages we'll delve into what some of these key man skills are, but right now let's look at one of the most important skills, as it's a huge part of one of our steps – **Alpha Nutrition** – and that's **cooking**.

THE ALPHA COOKING SCHOOL

We live in an age of mass convenience, which allows one to never even boil a kettle let alone cook a feast worthy of the Alpha buried deep inside of you. However, that sheep of convenience and purveyor of laziness isn't us. For you to have real game, be in great shape, and have real control over your diet you have to be able to cook, and cook well.

This is often not something we're taught as we grow up, unless we specifically take an interest in it. You may have watched your parents, paid attention and learned, or you may have taken no interest whatsoever. Regardless, you're now a man and being able to cook for yourself and others is a must-have skill.

We weren't all born wearing an apron, but it's never too late to learn <=== tweet that shit! @mcampbell2012 #UnleashYourAlpha

THE MAIN SKILLS EVERY MAN SHOULD POSSESS IN THE KITCHEN

The most important thing you must be able to do is read. This doesn't mean a piece of Russian literature, just lists and instructions. Once you have that nailed down, then you must be able to follow these instructions. You'll need to kickstart a desire to ensure you eat quality food and provide that for people close to you, will cement it.

If you can do these three things well then you can do anything related to the kitchen and cooking, from the most complex of dishes to the most mundane, but easiest tasks like boiling eggs.

Of course, it's not necessary to follow a recipe to the letter. There are many great resources out there for blokes of any level or experience, so if you have little or no clue, make an investment and buy a cookbook (I recommend more 'Paleo' style books, purely to ensure the recipes aren't flogged with nasty ingredients). *Healthy Everyday* by Pete Evans and Jamie Oliver's *My Guide To Making You A Better Cook* says it all. However, you'll find all your recipes from the menu plans referred to in this book in *'The Alpha Cook Book 2.0'*, downloadable with your bonus materials.

If you follow instructions you're most of the way there. We're going to cover some basic skills and behaviours below, but the main thing to realise is that cooking isn't hard nor should it be hard. Sure, there are some dishes that require real skill and expertise, but for our purposes you don't need to be in the same area code as them.

Here is a list of your basic requirements for cooking and kitchen know-how. Some of these are self-explanatory; others need more detail, which is all in *The Alpha Cook Book*. Read through and soak it up.

Cooking and kitchen must haves:

- Following a recipe is foolproof and vital.
- Know how to cook <u>at least</u> three dishes very well, and at least 5 passable meals.
- Cook the perfect steak.
- Know how to whip up a simple yet delicious salad and dressing.
- Be familiar with different meats (animals and cuts) and how to cut and cook them.
- Have 3 meat marinades/sauces and the ingredients for each marinade stocked.
- Know how to cook eggs 5 ways – boiling, poaching, scrambled, omelette, and fried.
- Understand the best ways to cook vegetables for nutrition, taste and time.
- Know how to use herbs, spices and seasoning to increase flavour and nutrition.
- Be familiar with which oils and fats to use and when.
- Master how to cook a breakfast fry up.
- Have one monster nutritious smoothie recipe.
- Know how to counter alcohol over indulgence.
- Be familiar with how to handle meats, vegetables, fruits.
- Learn the appropriate short cuts in the kitchen.
- Learn how to sharpen a knife.
- Know how to operate a BBQ, both gas and charcoal.

- Be mindful of others tastes, intolerances, and allergies.
- Know how to read food labels and what to look out for.
- Know where and how to shop.
- Understand how to clean up properly.

If you're lacking on many of these, then you need some work! The good news for you is mastering these things isn't hard. You should be able to smash these in no time and have them cemented as part of your new Alpha skills.

Get down to the supermarket or butcher and grocer, buy some nutritious food and get cooking. Start cooking for others, test things out and see what hits the mark. Remember this isn't just for you. Sure, you need to be a huge fan of your own cooking, but winning other people over with it puts you in true Alpha territory.

Read the details in your bonus material, find your strong and weak points. This is very important as most of us stick to the strong areas and avoid the weak ones. It may help you nail a few dishes but it won't do anything in the long run towards adding variety to your cooking and diet. Plus, this is great comfort zone breaking stuff.

***

Next come the other man skills. These are the attributes, know-how and behaviours that every man should *just know*. This is when you bring out your *Inner 007*. If you have these down, then awesome. Go save a cat stuck up a tree, or fix your own shirt. If not, get working on them – you never know when life is going to thrust you in the face of danger, potential embarrassment, or a likely man-brand maker of a situation.

ESSENTIAL ALPHA MAN SKILLS

- Be an awesome friend – stay in regular touch, get the first round, learn to recognise when your mates need help, go the extra mile for them, do what's needed.
- Be an even better lover. If you're getting intimate with someone then damn well get it right!
- Know how to wingman effectively.
- Make a woman melt in your arms with a kiss and give an awesome hug.
- Know how to give a decent massage.
- Know which flowers to buy and for what occasion. (Women **love** flowers.)
- Know how to make one cocktail well.
- Pour a beer with the perfect head.
- Always have a nice bottle of white wine in the fridge and a red in the cupboard.
- Know the birthdays of the people that matter and always wish them a happy one.
- Know how to give a decent handshake and always use someone's name.
- Know how to give basic CPR.
- Read and navigate a map.
- Know how to light a fire, hunt/catch/pick food, find water and make shelter in the wilderness.
- Be able to split firewood.
- Know how to catch, gut, and fillet fish.
- Know how to swim any stroke that will get you out of danger.
- Know how to climb a tree/rescue a cat stuck in a tree.
- Know how to grow vegetables and raise an animal for food.

- Carve a roast.
- Know how to iron a shirt and sew a button.
- Know how to dress for the occasion.
- Tie a tie.
- Do your laundry properly.
- Shuffle a deck of cards.
- Be able to nail the parallel park, back a trailer, change a tyre, jumpstart a car.
- Tell at least one awesome joke or story. People should be on the edge of their seat and want to share it.
- The ability to crank it – party hard when appropriate.
- It's fundamental to have a sense of humour and be able to laugh at yourself.
- Be a good listener.
- Open and eager to expanding your horizons by reading and intellectual discussions (without taking offence).
- Train like a beast – Squat at least 1.5x body weight, dead lift 1.75x body weight, bench press, chin-up and dip 1.25x body weight, military press 0.75x body weight.

Think I've missed some? Drop a comment on my Facebook page (**www.facebook.com/unleashyouralpha**) and add your suggestion.

CASE STUDIES

UNLEASH YOUR ALPHA CASE STUDIES

"A man with confidence is a man that will know how to take charge of his life."

– WILL HAUSERMAN

For this book I took on two case studies to show you how the methods and step-by-step guidelines work. Introducing, *Drew and Will.*

They were both in need of shedding some extra kilos, however, they were both also in need of some change and refocusing. They could both see things deteriorating in many aspects of their lives, so it was far more than just "weight loss" for these boys – it was getting back the control of their lives, gaining respect from partners or potentials.

They both showed body composition that was in "normal ranges," however, as time progressed it had been getting worse and the way things were going with work and other key lifestyle factors, it was a case of act now or see the little extra fat potentially become obesity and potential disease in 15 years.

These boys both applied for this position. They wrote a letter (Just as you will do for yourself – refer to page 55) explaining why they wanted this, how they were best suited for it, and how they were ready to make a change, because, they feared what would eventuate for them if they did not evolve.

It was a tough decision – there were a number of great applications, but I gradually managed to dwindle the list down to Drew and Will. We kicked things off 3 weeks before Christmas, looking at a 10-week intensive program following the tasks and key steps laid out in this book.

If you're thinking this process might be tough, then these boys can provide some insight about what they felt prior to the program and then what they were experiencing as we started the program and moved through to finish the process.

WILL

BEFORE

Stemming from some lengthy periods of inactivity and being 37 years old, I'm in the downward curve of middle-agedness; this includes a loss of direction and mental edge that could have been prevented. I know it's essential that these elements need to be in good order for life fulfilment on a day-to-day basis and beyond.

I've never reached a goal of significant note due to motivation slippage. I guess you could say with signs of early results, I take the foot off the throttle too soon.

I'm not going to lie, I love a pie and a beer. Though history shows, when required, I can go cold turkey on these indulgences. It's not these indulgences that cause me to break my regimes, it's always my exercise routine that breaks first each time.

I'm looking for the catalyst to turn my life around so I can look forward to the future. I could be on target to reach a life goal once and for all.

For too long now, I've been unhappy with my body and what I deem to be the most stubborn of fat layers in the midsection. I feel that with the realisation of reaching a physical goal for the first time, I'd gain a perspective on life that says anything can be achieved. So, any opportunity to first achieve this goal will no doubt flow on to achievements in relationships and career goals.

I had been accepting the softer layer around my midsection like I have been accepting my non-progressive position professionally and in other lifestyle areas. I maintained constant levels of lethargy and lack of zest across multiple areas of my lifestyle.

With a lifetime of goal setting not being an aspect of my psyche, I was always going to find this area of the course a challenge.

AFTER

To read Mike's description of a true Alpha is to simply describe the changes that occurred in me during the transformation process. I have definitely developed most of these attributes significantly.

If I want something, I am more likely than ever to go out and get it, or at least try to make it happen.

I now know that to be the real 'me', I need to be happy, and to be happy I need to be doing the things that I like doing. There is a focus and a confidence in me to go out and ensure that these things will get done. I always believed in my core values before the transformation and still believe in them. I will now be sure to apply them to more situations earlier so I don't allow these values to be compromised by a situation, relationship or environment in the future.

I never ever felt I was unhealthy before the transformation, but I never ever realised that I could feel so healthy and fit.

Furthermore, I feel stronger, more energised and most importantly positive about most things, most of the time. This is a big change to the man that applied for Mike's transformation process. The ability to be positive is the greatest gift I earned from the 10 weeks.

Mike's transformation has started me down a much better path and provided me with the basis of tools to continue to improve. These will also enable me to check-in with my existing lifestyle practices in the future to ensure that I am at a level or meeting an expectation that I have set for myself. Meeting my set targets and expectations will build happiness, and therefore, definitely result in confidence.

I know from the experience of the 10-week programme that anything is achievable and if you want something enough you can make it happen.

WILL'S STATS

VITAL STATISTICS	BMD*	TOTAL MASS**	TOTAL FAT MASS	TOTAL LEAN MASS	BODY FAT %
Before	1.227	93.4kg	13.5kg	76.7kg	14.5%
After (10 weeks)	1.263	88.3kg	8.4kg	76.6kg	9.5%
Change	+0.036	-5.1kg	-5.1kg	-0.1kg	-5%

* BMD- Bone Mineral Density in grams per cm squared g/cm²

** Measurements in kg

BEFORE AND AFTER

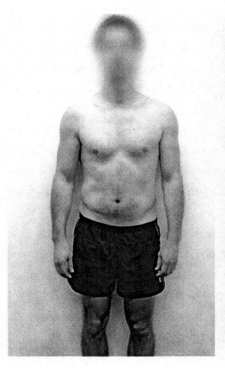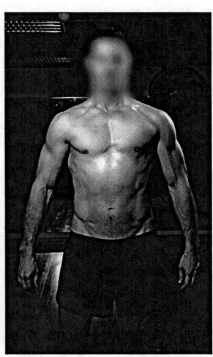

DREW

The application letter required me to evaluate aspects of my life, and understand what was required to improve my general health and well being. Drafting the initial letter made me recognise how unmotivated I had become to eat, drink, train and live with my future health in mind.

For the last seven years my career has been extremely demanding. Instead of prioritising my well-being, I ignored it and focused on my professional career. In the last 24 months, especially, I've noticed a decline in my physical health. The long hours in the office, constant travel and decline in motivation to exercise has resulted in additional weight gain and poor work life balance.

I found that my excess weight had caused other health problems that include: poor posture, regular aches and pains in my lower back, and poor recovery from exercise. All of these issues are weight related and are indicative of a lack of respect towards my body.

I've always been motivated to achieve academic goals but now I wanted to achieve personal lifestyle goals and correct old habits, to make some material changes. I would like to make some material changes to my life style and well being. I had accepted the status quo for too long and it was time to make changes to improve my personal and mental state.

The program was scheduled for ten weeks over the Christmas/New Year period, and required immense diligence and self-control. Changing habits is always difficult; however, the chosen period of time compelled me to reassess my exercise and well being while most people choose to over indulge and treat their bodies like an amusement park. Needless to say, I started the program with nervous excitement.

My weekly training regime required me to balance both work and training commitments. Training during normal business hours was difficult, however, on numerous occasions I stepped out of this shadow and took charge of the situation, training when I needed to, ensuring I still got my work done. Mike's guidance was instrumental here

The changes to my body shape were much greater than I anticipated and have set a benchmark for me to maintain in the future.

After making the initial adjustments to my diet and effectively managing my recovery, the program became easier. My key learnings included:

- *Making small and daily incremental changes was essential to implementing a sustainable regime.*
- *Structuring meals and training to be enjoyable.*
- *Understanding what exercises are required to ensure training is effective.*
- *Being held accountable by someone will improve my diligence to train and maintain a greater nutritional focus.*

The primary challenge during the program was a lack of support and understanding from people as to why I needed to make changes, and why I had chosen a period during the festive season to do so. After a physical change became apparent, those who initially queried the regime wanted to learn about the program. It was at this point that I realised the significance of the changes I'd implemented.

Mike has provided a suite of skills and tools for me to maintain a healthier approach to life. I have a greater respect for my health and wellbeing, in particular the food and meal portions I consume.

During the regime, Mike provided me with his definition of a true Alpha. I felt that I had many of the attributes prior to the program but I had neglected to apply them. Ultimately, I lacked motivation to focus on my own health, fitness and wellbeing. The program gave me the opportunity to revisit concepts I had stopped considering and reconcile what I need to do to be a better person.

It was not until I took time to reflect on my habits that I realised I could improve many aspects on my life. I definitely recommend the process.

DREW'S STATS

VITAL STATISTICS	BMD*	TOTAL MASS**	TOTAL FAT MASS	TOTAL LEAN MASS	BODY FAT %
Before	1.207	98.7kg	15.5kg	80.2kg	15.6%
After (10 weeks)	1.273	96.4kg	11.8kg	81.4kg	12.2%
Change	+0.066	-1.4kg	-3.7kg	+1.2kg	-3.4%

BEFORE AND AFTER

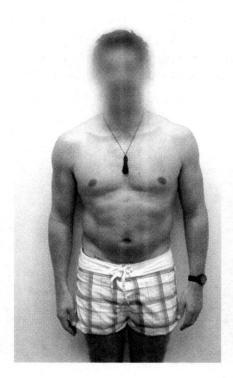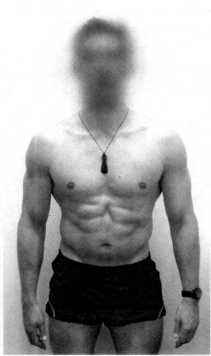

These two boys made such awesome progress in just 10 weeks, but the key to them doing so well was that they brought into the process and committed to themselves. They put their trust in the program, worked their butts off and then reaped the rewards.

These boys aren't freaks. They are normal guys, just like you and they proved, again, the effectiveness of this process. They proved that you can change your body, health, and life if you *really* want to, to, provided you have the correct information and guidance.

If you'd like to try a more hands on approach to this process rather than going through the steps in this book, turn to the back and you'll find out the various ways to take this further.

GO FORTH AND LEAD, MAN

THE INNER ALPHA WRAP UP

"If you can't fly then run, if you can't run then walk, if you can't walk then crawl, but whatever you do you have to keep moving forward."

– MARTIN LUTHER KING JR.

Initially, the aim of this book was to provide any man that reads it with a snappy, yet complete guide to getting your shit sorted and becoming a man that you're proud of, and who people respect. As I wrote (and wrote and wrote) the words flowed and I uncovered even more of the message that was inside me.

My experience and research over the last decade shows that the same issues and problems continue to reoccur – too often. Experts in mens issues and mental health confirm that the state of today's men is in a bad way and dwindling. Statistics show we are overweight, lacking in confidence and face depression at worrying rates. It seems, on the whole, we are incredibly unhealthy and lack the positive identity and balls we should have as men.

Forget the stats for a moment and just look around you. *We're not looking so good.*

We need a change and we need it now.

Reading this book and following all the steps isn't going to save *every* man from *any* life situation, but it sure will put you in an awesome place; looking great, feeling even better, stacked full of confidence with some real control in your life and drive for each day previously reserved for Facebook motivational quotes.

This is you finding your A-game and unleashing your inner Alpha. This is you becoming the best man you can be and reaping the rewards. This is you becoming a legend.

***

Not *every* guy is at anti-Alpha ground zero, but many of us have an area that needs work – some of us have many areas! That's exactly what this book is for, to be able to help any man that has something missing in his life to figure out what that is, and drive home a solution, a *long term* solution.

Of course we all have bad days, weeks, even months, however, if you're aware of these things, and you are actively working to improve yourself; including staying sharp, keeping control, remaining fit and healthy, then you'll be putting your best foot forward each day, no matter what level that's at.

We must always endeavour to move forward and be better men. This kind of attitude and approach to each day is what makes: great men, leaders, partners, friends and everyday Alphas. That's how you'll create and live a great life and how you'll inspire and help others to do the same.

You might be saying to yourself that getting in shape and eating well doesn't really seem like world changing stuff. However, that's *exactly* what it is. What this world needs is a new breed of man, a combination of the great parts of modern man with all the primal (and largely missing) parts of our ancestors.

"Don't ask what the world needs. Ask what makes you come alive, and go do it. Because what the world needs is people who have come alive."

– HOWARD THURMAN

Training and eating well are two of the very foundations that make a great man. These things help you develop your strength and confidence and go on to do great things, regardless of the scale.

As we've seen, for this to happen your head must be in the right place and you have to think. Putting concentrated time and effort into who you are, what you want out of each individual day and how you want to be perceived is critical. Asking yourself what your ultimate driver is and what ultimately makes you happy is vital for a man to be a real Alpha, *our Alpha*. Remember, it's the thoughts that lead to actions, and these actions become habits and soon this is who you are.

It's really quite simple when you set it out, so go back through the key points and start using your head.

***

Next comes the biggest factor – your nutrition. Getting this wrong can be a health, waistline, and libido killer. Having a fat gut and finding it harder to walk up a few flights of stairs is really only the start of a cascade of issues including low sex drive, diabetes, heart disease, depression and low confidence.

It's easy to see how so many can get it wrong; *mass advertising*, *feeble government policies*, *celebrity fads* and the know-it-all at work all present conflicting messages. It can be too much to even contemplate, let alone master.

However, it's really quite simple. When nailed on a regular

basis, *Alpha Nutrition* can be your best form of medicine and help to create the awesome body that that your mirror will reflect. Not to mention, *Alpha Nutrition* will shape a healthy, confident, and vibrant guy who loves each day.

Go through your key steps, soak it up, and attempt to write your own weekly meal plan. After that, check your appendix for the plans provided as well as your bonus material for more details and information.

For the most part you can follow the plans laid out in this book – pay attention to the food you eat and how your body reacts to it and let this be your guide. Once you've followed the guidelines and you're feeling awesome and starting to look like the kind of man you want to be, then you can start getting specific. In this instance, turn to the back to see how you can contact Mike if you have questions or would like guidance.

***

It's easy to see how exercise and training becomes so damn confusing for people. Sure, there aren't nearly as many differing opinions and in-your-face adverts trying to sway you as there are with food. However, because exercise (and getting to a point where you look good naked) involve hard work, people commonly look for an easy option – a quick fix.

This can lead to stagnation, frustration, injury, weight gain and a feeling of losing heart with training entirely. This often results in giving up until you reach breaking point (again) and feel you *need* to do something or you'll keep getting worse. Perhaps you're in danger of not having that realisation.

That's where the good news comes in. Training isn't that complicated – in fact it's really basic. You just have to work hard. There are *many* programs and philosophies, but if you stick to these principles and combine it with the other steps in this process, you'll be well on your way to becoming a ripped and athletic Alpha.

Again, go through your key points. Check the information in your bonus material if you want to learn about it, and then hit the programs.

Too many guys over think training and try to get all the details exactly right, constantly searching for *the* program that will finally get them in shape. Keep it simple and train as if you're an athlete and your paycheck depends on it. Take this on board:

"If you have a body, you are an athlete"

- BILL BOWERMAN

Always remember that, no matter who you are, where you live, or how old you are, you can train hard and get in shape.

***

Living a life that has balance in all areas often seems like some far off land. A time you might get to when you retire. However, it's that attitude and approach that will always prevent you from reaching it.

Many men today struggle with this concept of balance. We have too many hours at the office, not enough doing the things we enjoy with the people we enjoy, and not nearly enough quality sleep. The week can't go fast enough and the weekend is always too quick.

This pattern of high stress, little enjoyment, and poor sleep results in a vicious hormonal storm that, left unaltered, will lead to something I like to call *"pin the tail on the chronic illness,"* or *"disease roulette"*. Either way you're heading to a bad place.

One of the best tools for feeling amazing every day is managing stress by getting enough quality sleep. Many fatally underrate this, and this is why we have so many stressed out, fat and hormonally stuffed men everywhere.

Like everything so far, it doesn't have to be that way. There are some simple strategies you can put in place to ensure that you start to get more quality sleep, have less stress, and more enjoyment each day.

Some of this will start in our initial step of thinking and ensuring you have a positive frame of mind. Once you set some goals and focus them around your core values, you'll start heading in that direction each day. From there, food and training will impact hugely and then you can follow the steps to the life of a content and balanced man.

If this seems like 'a nice idea, but just isn't practical', then you *need* to sit down and get a check on your priorities. Go back to your core values and find out what matters most to you. If it's earning heaps and heaps of money so you have a big bank account and die rich, then fine, do so. However, if you want to spend time with your loved ones, doing things that give life meaning and make you smile, then re-jig your priorities and take control of your life. After all, this is what we're talking about – our Alpha has control of his life, not only that, *but he loves his life*.

***

The final step in your journey to unleash your Alpha is to master the finer points, the icing on the cake and the polish that makes the shoe shine. This is an area that gets lost on a lot of men and it shows in their refinement. Without consideration of the consequences of your choices and the external representation of your brand as a man, you'll be lacking when it comes to nailing the moments in life that matter.

No doubt, confidence will come from getting in shape, but it also comes from your actions, and you have to actively seek it and to improve your confidence levels and exude confidence.

We're not talking about arrogance, self-importance and selfishness. We're talking about subtle confidence, self-worth and looking after number one. We're also talking about being able to do the things that a man should do, like strolling the beach with his shirt off.

We've seen the missing link in our development with a lack of traditional rite of passage; this arguably causes us to enter a feminine dominant world missing out on the adequate influence of crucial masculine qualities. Or conversely, we have far too much masculine energy and we fall into a world of ego and macho bravado. Our primal and animal instincts are to garner respect and desirability in our society that encourages potential mates want to, well, mate with us. These instincts are losing traction as a result of our lifestyles, and it needs to be addressed by you for the Alpha male to walk proudly, more frequently in our world. This is what being an Alpha means.

This is exactly where the finer points of being an Alpha male are relevant. So, take note and start implementing the key elements of your *man skills* section.

Make sure you study the **Inner Alpha cooking and kitchen must haves** and start mastering the preparation of your own food. You don't have to fall in love with cooking, but you have to be able to be in charge of your nutrition.

Once you've started to initiate some of these steps and slowly mastered them, you'll see your confidence grow, your game improve, and things will start to happen in your life. This isn't due to the universe aligning for you, but because you're starting to develop a clear on yourself and becoming a better man. You'll be doing things for yourself. You'll be doing things for others. You'll be hustling all the time to improve and be an awesome guy – an Alpha legend.

Once you nail this stuff, then you can seek fine-tuning from a quality coach.

***

"The finish line is the start of a whole new race"

- UNKNOWN

I've been lucky enough to have some amazing coaches and mentors myself and I've learnt some awesome and invaluable life experiences from these mentors. Many of these insights you are reading in this book. However, two I haven't covered, and ones that have only really cemented themselves in the last 24 months or so are:

Be prolific, not perfect

and

Work your hustle muscle

To become an Alpha legend, a leader, a "people and great things magnet" and our Alpha, you have to be prolific with all things you do. Don't wait to perfect things or you'll miss opportunities. Get them to a point at which you're happy and get cracking. If need be, you'll iron out the wrinkles as you go.

If you're prolific, you're producing and if you're producing you're moving forward. This coincides or relates to hustle. To improve in any way, be it; losing body fat, advancing your career, getting laid, or simply getting to bed at a decent hour and waking refreshed – then you have to hustle and work your arse off. No one will do the big things for you – you have to take ownership of your own life, your own fate and hustle constantly.

You're now actively working to build your muscles and become strong. Well, you have to include one more: *your hustle muscle S*tart being prolific and increasing your hustle. Stop obsessing over the things that don't matter and just start doing. Get out beyond your comfort zone, stretch yourself and evolve. Make your own luck, remember.

"I build the road and the road builds me"

– AFRICAN PROVERB

This is about recognising the potential within you. This is about patience, practise, progression, and being prolific. This is about having maturity when it's needed and then laughing when it's not. This is about having a mission to become a better man and positively affecting the world and other people every day. This is about hustle and hard work. This is about building a better version of yourself – a great body, a great character, and a greater life. This is about being lit up in the morning and having a passion that sends you out the door so you continue to evolve and start kicking goals left, right and centre. This is about becoming more awesome, becoming a legend and an Alpha.

This is about becoming the perfect combination of James Bond, the great Nelson Mandela and Batman.

This is about becoming the man you were born to be.

This is your time to take life by the balls and start getting what you want out of it. *It's time to live man.* Your inner Alpha, your happiness and the things you really want await you.

Go and get them.

APPENDIX

THE SHREDDED ALPHA

FAT LOSS NUTRITION FOR A REAL MAN

A six-pack of abs may be sculpted in the gym,
but they're made in the kitchen.

Not every man wants a visible six-pack, which is fine. Most men want to "lose some of the fat from around the belly". (And if you have excess belly fat but don't want to lose it – *sort your shit out*).

This is very common – they just want to look lean and have the confidence that comes with looking great, both *with* clothes on *and* without. This alone can take men from anywhere from small wins on the anti-Alpha spectrum to kicking goals in every aspect of their lives, developing into fit, secure and athletic guys who are on top of their game.

For this to happen, we **must** address nutrition and we must do some things differently to the man who wants to be a professional athlete or simply "get massive." Seeing as most guys want to, and could do with, losing fat this is where we'll focus most of our energy. As you'll see later on, building muscle doesn't take too much tweaking.

When you have all the basics implemented, as outlined earlier, you will be well on your way to becoming our shredded Alpha. Once you have these down, then we will start to get specific in order to really help you get lean.

The next steps are:

Step 1: being prepared
Step 2: meal timings and content
Step 3: serving size
Step 4: have back up plans
Step 5: having a weekly 'relaxed meal'
Step 6: knowing how to fall off the wagon

**Go to your bonus nutrition material for much more detail involving these steps.

STEP 1: PREPARATION

No matter what your nutrition goals, being prepared is a must. This means either having your meals made and ready to go or knowing exactly where you will be getting your meals from.

For this we need strategies. We want Alpha kitchen efficiency – cooking on a time shoestring.

Protein is going to be a big part of your breakfast, so having extra meat in the fridge ready to eat is an easy and awesome preparation strategy. Another great technique is to cook something even larger, a boneless rolled leg of lamb for example. This might be 1 kilo of meat (or more), perfect. Cook the entire roast, eat your serving (roughly the size of your closed fist) and the rest can be used for meals the following day and breakfast beyond.

"The better prepared you are, the better position you are in to achieve your results" <=== Tweet that shit! @mcampbell2012 #UnleashYourAlpha

The other option is to buy your meals ready to go. If you are going to do this then you **must ensure** that the ingredients they use are in line with what you need on your journey to being our shredded Alpha. As we've discussed with buying ingredients, such as meat, you need to ask these questions. **Do not leave this up to the money saving tactics of a restaurant or takeaway food court style eatery.** Simply ask them what's in the dish you want to order and if it's full of processed sugar, vegetable oils, poor meat and other nasties then you will have to find somewhere new to eat.

If you're going to take the easy option of buying your food made for you and not put in the little effort to prepare your own, then you **must** put in the effort to make sure it's only quality ingredients.

Plan, prepare and prosper.

STEP 2: MEAL TIMINGS AND CONTENT

As with preparation, this is one of the major parts of any nutritional plan. There are many ideas out there and most of them have some sense and logical reason to them. However, many of them also contradict each other. Let's keep it very simple:

- Start by eating breakfast every day. As I alluded to above, this is going to largely contain quality protein, greens, and fats. Check your meal plans later for specific details.
- Everyone has a different metabolism, which responds in their own way not only to different foods, but to timing as well. You might operate better by only eating 2 big meals each day as opposed to someone who responds

better to 5 or 6 smaller ones, both containing the same amount of food.

There are no hard and fast rules – you must simply spread the food over the day in a manner which suits *you* and *your* body.

For the content make up of each meal you're going to ensure you get quality protein, greens and coloured veggies in **every meal.**

Food timing around training is important too. After your workout you need to ingest some protein and a small amount of quick acting carbs from fruit or honey. This protein hit might be from a shake. This will depend on when you train relative to your meal times or you might go straight for a meal of solid food.

Either way, within the first 45 minutes of completing the workout have one of these options. The sugar from the fruit will help promote the uptake of glucose and protein into your muscles, including key amino acid building blocks.

STEP 3: SERVING SIZES

As we've just seen, your serving sizes are going to depend directly on the frequency of your meals. Start noting down in your food diary how you felt after each meal. Were you full or satisfied? Paying attention to this stuff and knowing how your body responds to food is so crucial, yet it's also a very simple way to know your own body. **Eat slowly, until satisfied, not stuffed.**

STEP 4: ALWAYS HAVE A SLEEVE FULL OF BACK-UP PLANS

This is really re-enforcing the importance of being prepared. A back-up plan ensures that you don't fall into traps like going a full workday without eating due to a crazy schedule and then get some fast food. Back-up plans need to be up your sleeve and ready to take the place of plan A – normal shredded Alpha nutrition – when plan A either falls through or can't happen.

Get to know the food places around your home and work. You need to know where you can go if you've got literally no time to make dinner, or if you've played an away game and need to get breakfast on the way to work. Where can you get an omelette with bacon and spinach on the way to your work place?

In addition to this, there are things like meetings going on longer than planned. There's usually sweet treats, muffins, cakes, maybe sandwiches. This stuff is all going to derail your progress, especially if it happens often. Take in some nuts and fruit, or don't eat until after the meeting. Take control of your nutrition and don't cave to bullshit social pressures – that is not Alpha!

STEP 5: INCLUDE WEEKLY 'RELAXED MEALS'

You may have heard of the terms *cheat meals* and *cheat days*. Right now, for us, cheat meals are out and instead you'll be using *relaxed meals*.

The difference being that relaxed meals are still going to have an element of this entire plan to them, they're just more relaxed. If you desperately want to have a piece of toast with your eggs, bacon and spinach while out for breakfast at a cafe on Sunday, then do it. If you want to include a small dessert of gelato after dinner one night, then have at it.

These can be scheduled or not, but the key is to allow yourself these more relaxed meals. You're going to start with one per week maximum.

You'll note the two examples I gave aren't extreme – we're not talking about pigging out on pizza and beer or having a bowl of CocoPops with white sugar and low-fat milk. These don't fall remotely close to your guidelines and new nutritional plan. They are flat-out shitty meals – avoid them.

More "re-feed" type meals are for a later and more advanced time, but the odd bit of bread here and there for example, isn't the end of the world.

STEP 6: KNOWING HOW TO FALL OFF THE WAGON

This might sound counterintuitive, however, one thing we all do is fall off the wagon from time to time. It's a normal part of being human.

We all falter and have a bad meal sometimes. Gluttony takes over and you eat an entire pizza by yourself for lunch (for whatever reason – probably an emotional one). You need to make sure that is it, and not decide **Oh, I've blown out now; I may as well get back on track tomorrow.** This is a massive error of judgement, yet one that's so common and costly.

"The whole weekend was a right off, but I'll get back on track this week". This is so common it's painful. If you end up having a few beers on Friday night with the boys, then get back on track *that night!* Rehydrate, get a great sleep, and then make a quality breakfast the next day. Follow this up for the rest of

the weekend. Your willpower can be compared to your (soon to be) monster quads.

STEP 7: EAT A SALAD BEFORE YOU GO OUT (THIS ONE IS SELF-EXPLANATORY)

These key strategies are your blueprint for becoming our shredded Alpha. If you make them take the place of any current bad habits that don't align with these then you'll be on the road to being a fat loss success.

***

Now, let's take a look at my example week's shredded Alpha meal plan:

TIME	MONDAY	TUESDAY	WEDNESDAY	THURSDAY	FRIDAY	SATURDAY	SUNDAY
Breakfast ~ 6:30am	Turmeric & paprika chicken tenderloin & wilted spinach + handful nuts	**Turmeric & paprika chicken tenderloin & wilted spinach + handful nuts	**Turmeric & paprika chicken tenderloin & wilted spinach + handful nuts	Cinnamon & cacao protein yogurt with nuts & berries + boiled egg & greens drink	Cinnamon & cacao protein yogurt with nuts & berries + boiled egg & greens drink	Poached eggs & trout with fresh baby spinach, avocado and fried tomatoes	Omelette with bacon, avocado, wilted spinach & mushrooms
2nd Breaky ~ 10am	**1 Chinese 5 spice chicken thigh + spinach salad	**1 serving rump beef steak + Asian greens	**Turkey mince meatballs with mixed roast veggie salad	**1 serve of Moroccan lamb & Waldorf salad	**1 serve chicken, pumpkin, beetroot & feta salad	1 handful of nuts + 1 piece fruit	Cinnamon yogurt + berries & nuts
Lunch ~ 2pm	**1 Chinese 5 spice chicken thigh + spinach salad	**1 serving rump beef steak + roasted kumara & Asian greens	**Turkey mince meatballs with mixed roast veggie salad	**1 serve of Moroccan lamb & Waldorf salad	**1 serve chicken, pumpkin, beetroot & feta salad	1 piece chilli fillet steak on garlic kale + runny egg	Pork burger Pattie on open salad of lettuce, avo, tomato & beetroot/ kumara mash
2nd Lunch ~ 4pm	No meal	No meal	No meal	No meal	No meal	No meal	No meal
Dinner ~ 7:30pm	1 serving marinated rump beef steak + roasted kumara & Asian greens	Turkey mince meatballs with mixed roast veggie salad	1 serve of Moroccan lamb & Waldorf salad	1 serve chicken, pumpkin, beetroot & feta salad	1 medium piece of white fish + quinoa salad	'Relaxed meal' eg. Spicy tomato steamed mussels with sourdough + 'Alpha desert'	1 Chinese 5 spice chicken thigh + spinach salad
Post workout	1 x 30g scoop of WPI protein with water + 2 fresh dates	1 x 30g scoop of WPI protein with water + 1 banana	Rest day	1 x 30g scoop of WPI protein with water + 1 banana	1 x 30g scoop of WPI protein with water + banana	1 x 30g scoop of WPI protein with water + 2 fresh dates	Rest day

All recipes are in the downloadable '*The Alpha Cook Book*'

** = left over/prepared the night before or earlier in the week

These meals are all designed to be made yourself, but some of the weekend options you'll be able to get at many places. They might not be on the menu exactly like that, but simply ask to have it that way. For example, generally a cafe chef won't mind changing the order to include spinach instead of toast and so on.

Now get cracking into the recipes in the cookbook and follow this eating plan. It's easy and all of these meals are delicious and very nutrient dense – *exactly what we want!*

If you're still hungry, deal with it by having some veggies first, then protein and follow with fat. For example, a carrot and a boiled egg.

THE MUSCULAR ALPHA
NUTRITION FOR A GROWING MAN

"Eat big to get big"

When it comes to putting on muscular size and getting bigger, like anything with nutrition there are many ways to skin a cat. However, to save cats from losing their skin, we'll be sticking to a **very simple approach:**

MORE of the same

We've seen so far that regardless of your goals, you must be eating natural – whole, nutrient dense foods. To shed body fat, we eat these foods to a certain caloric intake. Exactly what number we don't need to worry about right now because it's too complicated and time consuming.

Do you want to spend hours going through charts, weighing food and calculating macro nutrient amounts? I'm going to guess no. The key is knowing your body, what it needs and eating slowly so you can manage the amount you eat and stop when you feel *satisfied*.

However, for those that want to put on muscle, you'll simply be eating a lot more of these quality calories. We'll also be adding in some fantastic calorific snacks and little techniques that will have your muscles in need of a bigger shirt.

Now, there are terms out there in the fitness world that are backwards and stupid. I could go on for a while and list them but the one we're interested in here is *"bulking"* (purely eating *anything* and everything to "get big'). This is in no way what you're going to be doing here.

I make no apologies here in saying this is unhealthy, uninformed, arduous, pointless, and dumb.

What we're going to be doing is increasing muscle mass while **dropping body fat** (or maintaining). Outrageous I know, but entirely doable once the right framework is followed and care is put into your nutrition. The two go hand in hand. The more muscle mass you have, the more your body will use fat for fuel, unless you "bulk." Not only this, but you'll also have better energy, a great sex drive, fertility, and mental health.

That means quality food options at each meal, in bigger portions and more frequently. There will be times that your content proportions change slightly, for example, you'll now be eating a lot more carbs than our shredded Alpha.

Let's follow our steps from the previous section and alter where need be.

STEP 1: PREPARATION

Nothing changes here except that you'll now be preparing more food.

STEP 2: MEAL TIMINGS AND CONTENT

To get big and put on some real muscular size you need to eat more, simple as that. You'll now be looking to eat at least 5 meals a day. This isn't absolutely necessary, but helps in getting the volume consumed (you can still try 2 meals but they'll have to be massive, and your digestion will struggle). The content will contain more of everything, especially carbs by proportion.

STEP 3: SERVING SIZE

This is, again, something that will take some amount of listening to your body, as we don't want you to eat and eat and eat until you can't digest a lot of the food, or worse, it causes some adverse reactions such as intolerances.

However, in saying that *you must overfeed your muscles.* Aim to have a large serving of protein each meal. For rough amounts try getting 1.5-2 fists per meal and up to 2-2.5 on heavy training days. Include plenty of leafy green vegetables and other vegetables (2 fists). Also include root vegetables as starchy carbs like kumara and pumpkin, or perhaps some quinoa or fruit (1-1.5 fist). Also include some quality fats (1 thumb).

And remember your first meal after training will be your

monster meal. For this meal, think about 2 closed fists worth of protein, about 3 fists worth of vegetables, and with that 1.5 fist of starchy vegetables, quinoa or rice. Remember to follow the aforementioned eating strategies to fine-tune *your* amounts.

STEP 4: STOCK YOUR SLEEVE FULL OF BACK UP PLANS

Again, get organised with a list of good places nearby. You need to eat a lot of food remember!

Snacks like nuts, raw veggies, and fruits alone won't cut it. Sure, you can get them on board, but we also want more solid protein and fats. For example, try having a jar of coconut butter at work for example and have a spoon full of it with nuts and some quality biltong – a delicious and a great muscle-building snack.

The other easy option here is a nutrient dense smoothie. Make this up and take it with you in a bottle or container and either consume throughout the day or have it as a back-up plan. You'll find this in the bonus cookbook.

STEP 5: INCLUDE A WEEKLY 'RELAXED MEAL'

This still applies, but can be somewhat more flexible in terms of its content. For example, you'll be adding in some more and different carb options. More of the same with more carbs, remember.

STEP 6: KNOWING HOW TO FALL OFF THE WAGON

Nothing changes here. Have faith in yourself long term and see the blip as exactly that, a minor scratch that you can relax about, but know you'll fix it by staying on track outside of that.

***

Let's take a look at the specifics. First, some great muscle building tricks, techniques, and snack options and then our example weekly food plan:

Tricks and snacks:

- Liquid calories are a great way to add to your overall intake, especially fats. For example, add butter to greens, extra virgin olive oil to salads, cook with extra virgin coconut oil every time you fry as well as adding this to smoothies. When you cook meat in the oven, remove some of the fatty juices and pour some over the meat when you dish it up. You'll thank me.
- With the right ingredients, smoothies and shakes can easily be sipped and added in as extra meals to really increase your overall count of quality calories.
- We've touched on this already, however, when you eat ensure that you're relaxed and taking your time. The reason? Stress and on-the-go eating means poor digestion. Relax, digest, and absorb.
- High protein snacks are very handy to have on hand. Biltong, shredded chicken, any meat, and boiled eggs are all fine options.
- Protein supplements are a must for the growing Alpha.

Whey protein isolate is ideal for post training, however, another gem to help muscle growth is using casein protein before bed. This is much slower releasing so it will aid in growth and muscular repair whilst you sleep. Try having a 30g scoop with 2 tablespoons of natural yogurt and a glass of full fat milk (or water).

Let's look at your sample weekly *muscular Alpha* nutrition plan. Remember, all recipes are in *The Alpha Cook Book*. This will also contain drinks, smoothies, and shakes. If you're up earlier just modify the times for yourself, but whatever you do – *start eating man!* Remember, you can eat fewer meals than in here, but they will have to be larger.

TIME	MONDAY	TUESDAY	WEDNESDAY	THURSDAY	FRIDAY	SATURDAY	SUNDAY
Breakfast ~ 6:30am	2 x Turmeric & paprika chicken thighs & wilted spinach + handful nuts	2 x Turmeric & paprika chicken thighs & wilted spinach + handful nuts	2 x Turmeric & paprika chicken thighs & wilted spinach + handful nuts	Fillet steak + garlic mushrooms + wilted spinach	Fillet steak + garlic mushrooms + wilted spinach	2 x Poached eggs & bacon with fresh baby spinach, avocado & fried tomatoes	Omelette with bacon, avocado, wilted spinach & mushrooms + sourdough
2nd Breaky ~ 10am	Alpha smoothie	** 1 serving curried prawns & quinoa	Alpha Smoothie	** 1 serve of easy roast chicken & veggies	**1 medium piece of white fish, greens + quinoa salad	Alpha smoothie	Cinnamon, WPI, yogurt + berries & nuts
Lunch ~ 1pm	** Butterflied lamb leg + Greek salad & duck fat roasted kumara	** 1 serving curried prawns & quinoa	**Pork loin medallions & celeriac slaw	** 1 serve of easy roast chicken & veggies	**1 medium piece of white fish, greens + quinoa salad	1 serving bacon Brussels sprouts & steak mix	Pork burger Pattie on open salad of lettuce, avo, tomato, beetroot & kumara mash
2nd Lunch ~ 4pm	** Butterflied lamb leg + Greek salad & duck fat roasted kumara	1 tbsp coconut butter + almonds + biltong	**Pork loin medallions & celeriac slaw	Boiled eggs & capsicum boats	Shaved turkey breast roll ups + boiled egg	1 tbsp coconut butter + almonds + WPI yogurt shake	1 tbsp coconut butter + almonds + biltong
Dinner ~ 7pm	1 serving curried prawns with quinoa	Pork loin medallions & celeriac slaw	1 serve of easy roast chicken & veggies (incl skin)	2 medium pieces of white fish Asian Greens + quinoa salad	Alpha chicken burgers + kumara fries	'Relaxed meal' e.g. Thai green curry & basmati rice + dessert	Butterflied lamb leg + Greek salad & duck fat roasted kumara
Pre-bed	WPI yogurt shake (or raw milk*)	Cinnamon, WPI, yogurt + berries & nuts	WPI yogurt shake (or milk*)	Cinnamon, WPI, yogurt + berries & nuts	WPI yogurt shake (or raw milk*)	No meal	No meal
Post workout	1 x 30g scoop of WPI protein with water + 4 fresh dates & banana	Alpha post workout smoothie deluxe	Rest day	Alpha post workout smoothie deluxe	1 x 30g scoop of WPI protein with coconut water + banana & honey	1 x 30g scoop of WPI protein with coconut water + 4 fresh dates	Rest day

** leftovers

* Refer to guidelines on milk for specific milk used here.

Get cracking into cooking these recipes and eating these meals. Your keys here are to keep the content quality and simply get more of the good stuff, especially protein and good carb options.

Remember, when you're out and about, if something doesn't fit the bill, then ask the waiter to slightly alter your order – you've got a right to control what goes in your mouth, so start doing it!

***

Go to your additional nutrition material to see a whole bonus section. **The All-round Alpha** section will give nutrition advice for the man who wants to maintain leanness, muscle mass, energy, have a great sex drive, and tip top mental health – *our Alpha.*

If you are confident in yourself, have great energy, health, fitness, strength, virility and you look like one masculine motherfucker, you, my friend, are the man.

This section contains another sample week meal plan, plus examples as well as strategies for the man who travels a lot. Nutrition tips for long holidays are covered too.

THE ALPHA SUPERFOODS

Now for the bonus nutritional tips that many people miss, which can have amazing benefits for anyone. Not only do these things add awesome flavour to meals but they are jammed packed full of nutritional goodness that help you flight oxidation, inflammation, and keep you healthy and lean.

There are a few foods we haven't mentioned yet, but they can be a strong weapon in the Alpha arsenal:

Herbs & spices – They have fat burning properties, help build muscle, and get your body operating better on a daily basis. Plus, they'll turn any plain meat dish into something you'll annoy friends about regaling for days.

There are many beneficial herbs & spices, but let's run through a few of the best:

- **Turmeric:** Has powerful natural anti-inflammatory properties as well as being an effective antioxidant. This alone makes turmeric a must-have for every modern man. Anything that will fight oxidative stress and systemic inflammation will help you with any health and body goal. Try using in smoothies, adding to marinades, or simply sprinkle on meat.

- **Cinnamon:** Cinnamon has been shown to regulate blood glucose, have a positive effect on cholesterol and inflammation. As well as being a tasty addition to many dishes, foods and recipes, cinnamon will move you closer to looking and feeling great.

- **Cumin:** Similar to the above, cumin has been linked with blood sugar regulation and fighting inflammation. Cumin also has antibacterial properties and aids in digestion by stimulating pancreatic enzyme secretion, which assists in the breakdown of food and absorption of nutrients.

- **Chilli & Cayenne pepper:** The potent ingredient capsaicin, combined with vitamin A, in these spicy powers act to improve health in a number of ways. This includes, fighting inflammation, stimulating the digestive tract and boosting immunity.

- **Paprika:** An awesome flavour addition to many things, paprika is high in vitamin C, which aids in healing, recovery, and iron absorption. It also contains capsaicin and has anti-inflammatory properties.

- **Nutmeg:** Another great addition to many dishes and meats, nutmeg also has a number of beneficial properties, including increasing circulation, calming muscle spasms, combating anxiety/tension, lowering blood pressure, and helping concentration.

- **Fennel:** A versatile vegetable with powerful seeds. Fennel seeds have been shown to help with the maintenance of bone. It has also been used for centuries as a digestive aid, while also having high iron content and potentially helping the body flush toxins.

- **Rock salt or sea salt:** Salt should have a colour to it – bland white table salt is processed rubbish like table sugar. These salts are not only crucial to the bodies normal functioning, but aid in optimal health. Have it on cooked foods or small amounts in water, so the vital trace minerals can aid the body in working efficiently and effectively. Oh, and it makes food taste awesome.
- **Black pepper:** Pepper is an awesome addition to most foods to enhance taste, however, it also aids in the uptake of other compounds into the body. It also contains manganese and vitamin k to help bone strength, making it a great addition to any meal.

Start getting these into your cooking, adding to meat and vegetables, and putting in smoothies. Basically wherever you can, get some super spices in!

Fermented foods – Sauerkraut (cabbage), kim-chi, carrots, beetroots, coconut flesh, quality yoghurt, kefir, products using liquid whey from raw milk, and products that contain live cultures to name a few. This stuff acts to aid gut health, digestion, and overall health. Try having a tablespoon before each meal.

Organ meats – Often the forgotten parts of animals, however, if the animal is healthy and naturally raised then their organs are a superpower of nutrients. The two I recommend most for nutrient power and versatility in cooking are liver and kidneys. Of course, that doesn't mean you should rule out eating some balls... This is often a real comfort zone breaker and conversation starter in the very least!

Bone broths and stocks – This means homemade, however, not necessarily by you. Many butchers and small deli-style stores sell homemade versions. Broths are packed with amazing nutrition and are a tremendous addition to any diet, be it shredding, gaining muscle, or just good health.

*To see Mike's video recipe of bone broth visit this link: **www.youtube.com/ watch?v=O7iJkRqqXgY***

To see Mike talk about these 'Alpha Superfoods' visit **www.youtube.com/ watch?v=XG4pFcyqG6s**

SUPPLEMENTATION
FILLING NUTRITIONAL HOLES

Because we largely live in a western society of immediate solutions and an "I want it now" mentality, the supplementation industry has been so successful because a large majority of people want a quick fix. So let's clear the air – **there are no quick fixes. Attaining fat loss, great body composition, and good health are continuous processes, which you must work at.**

Supplements won't provide a magic pill that will transform you into great health. What they will do is add to your great nutrition and provide a top-up in the areas that need a boost. Since many farming and production practices strip even our best foods of vital nutrients, it helps to be vigilant about adding them back in.

This is where supplementation comes in.

For full guides and descriptions, see your downloadable bonus *Alpha Supplementation Guide*.

The 8 key supplements every Alpha and aspiring Alpha should consider taking:

- **Wild fish oil or krill oil** (omega 3 fatty acids DHA and EPA) – breakfast and dinner.
- **Probiotic –** before breakfast.
- **Vitamin D –** Unless you live near the equator and spend your days in the sun, you need this.
- **Magnesium, zinc, B6 or ZMA –** before bed.
- **Powdered greens –** chlorella, spirulina, wheat grass, barley grass + 'extras'.
- **Whey protein Isolate (WPI) –** post workout at least.
- **Branch Chain Amino Acids (BCAAs) –** during heavy workouts.

The 5 supplements worth considering:

- **Digestive enzymes** – after meals.
- **Beta-Alanine –** pre workout in one dose or spread through day.
- **Vitamin C with bioflavonoids –** if run down.
- **Glutamine –** post workout.
- **Creatine monohydrate –** post workout.

Nutritional take home 20: Supplements are to be exactly that – *supplementary* to optimal nutrition. These are used to fill whichever gaps you can't fill with your diet and to help optimise your overall nutrition and lifestyle. The icing on the cake, so to speak.

Could you benefit from anything else? Quite likely, but that will require detailed blood and saliva analysis and skilled examination of the results.

If you feel fatigued a lot, suffer from bloating or experience an inability to recover, then you might need to dig deeper. In such cases, I recommend finding a quality naturopath or doctor and getting some tests done.

Feel free to email Mike with any questions as well. We deal with individual needs, such as these, within the Alpha online coaching.

WHERE TO FROM HERE?

Thanks for reading this book, it means a lot to me.

My in-person 12 week program (run with my team of experts) is an exclusive program for professional men. If you want to know more about the program, or how you can get involved, then contact me at **info@unleashyouralpha.com**

I also run my program via online coaching. To check out more about it and apply for a spot in the next intake visit **unleashyouralpha.com/online-coaching**

Outside of these two very hands-on coaching programs you can partake in my 'Beast-Gentleman-Legend 16 week challenge' group program which follows the principles and plans in this book but with group accountability plus support and coaching from me. To enquire email **info@unleashyouralpha.com**

Take the online 'Alpha Benchmark' test to see where you currently sit as a man, and get your opportunity to have a call with me to discuss the result. Visit: **unleashyouralpha.com/alpha-benchmark**

Join my email list to get free gifts and my best content to your inbox, visit **unleashyouralpha.com**

Please come and join the community on facebook at **facebook.com/unleashyouralpha**

And subscribe to my YouTube channel for all the latest videos at **youtube.com/user/unleashyouralpha**

Also, please feel free to visit **unleashyouralpha.com/book/book-bonus-materials** for more on the book and to find your *Bonus Material.*

My personal website **mikecampbelltraining.com** is also where you can find out more about me and how to work with me.

Visit **amazon.com** *and write a (ahem, favourable) review on this book you'll receive a free entry to either an in-person or Skype 'Alpha Benchmarking Session'. Write your review and email Mike to claim your ticket.*

ABOUT MIKE CAMPBELL

Mike is a trainer, coach, author and the ultimate food and training geek.

When he started as a personal trainer nearly 10 years ago, he didn't envisage coming across the same issues day in and day out, however, he did, and constantly has. Now he focuses on solving these problems for men, and also what led to him writing this book.

Mike is incredibly passionate about helping guys become the best man they can be. Mike is the mastermind and creator of the 'Unleash Your Alpha Program' – a proven system for helping men unleash the power and awesomeness that lies within them.

Plus he loves to cook, eat and talk to his food. He loves stone fruit, cold beer, red wine and to think of himself as a low level Batman. He likes to lift heavy things, eat a large variety of meat and write short bios.

You'll find his advice to be uncomplicated and immediately actionable. Mike believes strongly in making things easy to follow and implement and cutting out the confusing noise and misinformation in the health and fitness industry.

ACKNOWLEDGEMENTS

It's often one of those tired clichés – words can't express my gratitude – yet the fact that an author has just written it, makes it seem somewhat unbelievable. They are a writer, after all.

However, now that I'm here, facing writing thanks of my own in a book I've laboured over for quite some time, I am lacking words. I know that this doesn't speak of my inability to put it into words, more of the immense positive influence that this person has had on me. Nardia, you are simply an amazing person, a constant inspiration. You challenge me daily and without you in my life, these words would not exist. None of them, and none of it – the blogs, the book, the magazine covers, the growth and the profile. 'Meat' Mike Campbell would not be. To you, an infinite thank you's.

"She's my queen, my rock, my fire" .

Having set the tone of these thanks, let me bring it down somewhat, no offense intended at the following people, but you know, Nardia does other things too. Pretty hard to match that...

To my family; Dad, Liss, Ben, Kate, Craig and the little munchkins. You guys have been my biggest supporters and source of encouragement. You have always supported me to do what makes me happy. I can safely say I am now most definitely doing that, and of course am over the moon that I can now give advice back, sometimes ad nauseam... Liss and Ben, thank you so much for your proofing brilliance!

And, of course, the one painfully obvious missing part of our clan, mum. One of the true sparks for this journey, book, business, personal growth and drive to help others live a healthier and better life. Not a day goes by without me thinking of your smiling face, your strong grit and your wholehearted approach to life and your family. I love you always; you are a true inspiration to me.

To all of my clients past and present, thank you. Without you guys none of this would have ever come about for you are and have been my constant research team for close to a decade. My human guinea pigs and sounding boards- thank you.

To all of my friends who have in some way helped with this process, big or small, thank you. Special mention to Raph for your assistance, and to the boys for always keeping me on my toes, even if it does involve me getting shit for modelling on gay magazine covers. And Duncan for your endless accountability, ideas, feedback and support – it would have been a whole lot harder without you mate!

To the KPI community that not only created this and fostered it, but provided continual advice, ideas and support. One of the special networks of inspired and inspiring people I am truly grateful to be a part of. Dan and Glen, you guys have helped me find my compass, refine it and get shit done. Your skills, openness and inspiration has turned me into an advocate for life and a GSD machine. Much love. And to Andrew, the coach – the first day I spent with you, you put me at ease and 100% made me realise "I can do this". Thank you so much for the system. Look, this is my book – you did this! And Kylie, thanks for believing in me, you are a star!

To the two boys who featured in this book – Will and Drew. In a time when most are relaxing during the holiday period, sinking beers and over-eating, you showed that with some balls, determination and the right guidance, changing your body and making significant strides in your life is more than possible. You are two absolute weapons who made it through the 10 weeks (2 x Alphas unleashed!) and I thank you for not only putting your trust in me, but your ongoing support, cheers boys. And big thanks to Simon for shooting Will and providing the images; expert work, as always.

A massive thank you to all the people I interviewed for this book. It was a true honour to share a part of your private thoughts and opinions – in particular, Pete Evans, Dr Jonathan Phillips, Nathan Charles, John Broadbent, Andrew Creagh, Dr Elizabeth Celi and Pete Manuel. To the people I've quoted but never met, I clearly think you're a bit of alright... love your work, thank you!

To Julie and the team at OpenBook Creative, I am so grateful for your patience and calming presence, when the reality of getting words into an actual book seemed overwhelming, you were brilliant.

To others who had a special part in this in some way; Cassie, Paul, Jon. Jon you have helped me a lot over the last year. Your guidance and example has consistently showed me the way. And of course for introducing me to Bryan, who I must thank. To a man I've never met in person (we will rectify that someday soon), thank you for taking something so personal and close to me, and tearing out the superfluous and making it sound all the better. You are an artist and a gentleman. Thank you for the expert polish.

To every person who has replied, "Fuck yes, that's awesome, I love it!" when they've heard what I've been intent on writing about – thank you. That kind of thing may seem like a throw-away comment to you, but it fuels me to keep going.

To all the unknown blokes who I thought of when writing – this was designed to help you. No offence but I think you need this book, that's why I wrote it. To every guy who's tried and failed, to every 'weekend warrior', to every confused question I've ever had, to the guy that suits up every day and heads to work, does his thing and either complains about it after or suffers in silence – thank you. You have inspired me to address the everyday 'anti-alpha' problem and come up with a real solution to help every man become his best and live an awesome life.

Fat Freddy's Drop who, coincidently, or not really, also deserve a thanks. Your music was the soundtrack to my writing sessions.

Peace

And to me. Good shit brother!

Chur everyone!
Mike

REFERENCES

Collins dictionary online, http://www.collinsdictionary.com/

Oxford dictionary online, http://oxforddictionaries.com/

2012 WBI US Workplace Bullying, Survey,
http://www.workplacebullying.org/
    wbiresearch/2010-wbi-national-survey/

Australian Parliament Magazine, http://www.aph.gov.au/~/
    media/05%20About%20Parliament/53%20HoR/537%20
    About%20the%20House%20magazine/46/PDF/Poison1.
    ashx

Victorian Goverment, Australia- Better Health Channel:
    http://www.betterhealth.vic.gov.au/bhcv2/bhcarticles.nsf/
    pages/Domestic_violence_why_men_abuse_women
http://www.betterhealth.vic.gov.au/bhcv2/bhcarticles.nsf/
    pages/Hormones_cortisone

Leisl Mitchell , Parliament of Australia- Domestic violence in Australia—an overview of the issues: http://www.aph.gov.au/About_Parliament/Parliamentary_Departments/Parliamentary_Library/pubs/BN/2011-2012/DVAustralia

John Broadbent of *Man Unplugged*

Steve Biddolph, the author of *Raising Boys* and *The New Manhood*

David Deida *The Way Of The Superior Man*

The Fear of Losing Control- What's behind this fear and how you can overcome it, Elliot D. Cohen, Ph.D. http://www.psychologytoday.com/blog/what-would-aristotle-do/201105/the-fear-losing-control

John Romaniello & Adam Bornstein – *Engineering The Alpha*

The New England Journal of Medicine, The burden of disease and the changing task of medicine. David S. Jones, M.D., Ph.D., Scott H. Podolsky, M.D., and Jeremy A. Greene, M.D., Ph.D.- http://www.nejm.org/doi/full/10.1056/NEJMp1113569

Birth cohort trends in major depression: increasing rates and earlier onset in New Zealand , Peter R. Joyce et. al. Journal of Effective Disorders, http://www.sciencedirect.com/science/article/pii/016503279090063E

Peter McAlister- *Manthropology*

He'll Be Ok by Celia Lashlie

Good Calories Bad Calories by *Gary Taubes*

Australian Bureau of Statistics- Australian Health Survey
    2011-2012, http://www.abs.gov.au/ausstats/abs@.nsf/
    Lookup/4125.0main+features3330Jan%202013
http://www.abs.gov.au/ausstats/abs@.nsf/
    Lookup/4832.0.55.001main+features42007-08
http://www.abs.gov.au/ausstats/abs@.nsf/0/947114F16DC7D-
    980CA25773700169C64?opendocument
http://www.abs.gov.au/ausstats/abs@.nsf/
    Lookup/26DB864DADDA4011CA257AA30014BAA7
http://www.abs.gov.au/ausstats/abs@.nsf/
    Lookup/4D709A4E0614C546CA257AA30014BD06

Investigating alcohol-related violence, Australian catholic
    University, http://www.acu.edu.au/about_acu/our_uni-
    versity/newsroom/news/media_releases/repository/
    investigating_alcohol-related_violence

Australian Institute of Criminology

A Woman's Worth by Marianne Williamson

Serious Mental Illness Increases Risk Of Cancer And
    Injuries, Grace Rattue , Medical News Today- http://www.
    medicalnewstoday.com/articles/248101.php

Military must persevere to solve suicide issue, By Karen Parrish,
    Us Department of Defence- http://www.defense.gov/news/
    newsarticle.aspx?id=116571

Testosterone and men's health, *Journal of Behavioural Medicine, Booth A, Johnson DR, Granger DA*

Cortisol — Its Role in Stress, Inflammation, and Indications for Diet Therapy, By Dina Aronson, MS, RD, *Today's Dietitian,* Vol. 11 No. 11 P. 38)

Stephen Smith, http://www.articlesbase.com/health-articles/insulin-leptin-ghrelin-the-3-fat-hormones-933564.html

Matthew Fox, http://www.livestrong.com/article/371839-leptin-and-ghrelin-information/

The Relationship between Libido and Testosterone Levels in Aging Men, Thomas G. Travison, John E. Morley, Andre B. Araujo, Amy B. O'Donnell and John B. McKinlay, The Journal of Clinical Endocrinology and Metabolism, http://jcem.endojournals.org/content/91/7/2509.short

Impaired Insulin Signaling in Human Adipocytes After Experimental Sleep Restriction: A Randomized, Crossover Study; Josiane L. Broussard et al.

Role of Insulin Resistance in Human Disease, Gerald M Reaven, American Diabetes Association, http://diabetes.diabetes-journals.org/content/37/12/1595.short

Glucagon, Health Information from the National Library of Medicine, http://www.nlm.nih.gov/medlineplus/druginfo/meds/a682480.html

Testosterone and men's health, Booth A, Johnson DR, Granger DA, Journal of Behavioural Medicine, 1999; 1-19.

Estrogens in men: clinical implications for sexual function and the treatment of testosterone deficiency, Kacker R et. al. Journal of Sexual Medicine, 2012 Jun;9(6):1681-96, http://www.ncbi.nlm.nih.gov/pubmed/22512993

Hidden messages in water by Dr Masaru Emoto

Sport Nutrition by Michael Gleeson Asker Jeukendrup

John DeMartini http://masteryourlifepower.com/demartini-method-2/7-areas-of-life/

Myths And Truths About Soy from the *Weston A Price Foundation*- http://www.westonaprice.org/soy-alert/myths-and-truths-about-soy

http://www.realmilk.com/

Rob Williams, Organic Strength Development: How Strong is Strong Enough?

Examine.com – Supplement-Goals-Reference Guide, Sol Orwell and Kurtis Frank

http://stereopsis.com/flux/

Adrenal Fatigue: The 21st Century Stress Syndrome by James Wilson

The 5 Love Languages by Gary Chapman,
www.the5lovelanguages.com

The Benefit of Power Posing, Amy J. C. Cuddy,
Harvard Business School Working Paper, No. 13-027

The Urban Dictionary; http://www.urbandictionary.com/define.
php?term=bromance

Adapted cold shower as a potential treatment for depression,
Shevchuk NA, Med Hypothesese 2008;70(5):995-
1001. Epub 2007 Nov 13, http://www.ncbi.nlm.nih.gov/
pubmed/17993252

Immune system of cold-exposed and cold-adapted humans,
Janský L, Pospíšilová D, Honzová S, Ulicný B, Srámek
P, Zeman V, Kamínková J, European Journal of Applied
Physiolopy and Occupational Physiology. 1996;72(5-6):445-
50, http://www.ncbi.nlm.nih.gov/pubmed/8925815

Special thanks to the below for their interview input:

John Broadbent
Pete Manuel
Pete Evans
Dr Jonathan Phillips
Nathan Charles
Andrew Creagh
Dr Elizabeth Celi

Published in 2014 in Australia by Mike Campbell
mike@unleashyouralpha.com
www.unleashyouralpha.com

Text copyright © Mike Campbell 2014
Book Production: OpenBook Creative
Cover Design: OpenBook Creative
Editor: Brian Krahn
Photographer: Simon Lee

Australia Cataloguing-in-Publication entry:
Author: Mike Campbell
Title: Unleash Your Alpha : eat like a man, train like a beast,
operate like a gentleman & become a legend

9780987585301 (paperback)
9780987585325 (ebook : epub)
9780987585318 (ebook : kindle)

Subjects: Men - Life skills guides
Men - Psychology
Men - Conduct of life
Men - Health and hygiene
Self-actualization (Psychology)
Masculinity.

Dewey Number: 155.332

Disclaimer: This book is a source of general information only. This general information cannot, and does not, address your individual situation and so is not a substitute for the advice of a suitably qualified professional who knows your personal circumstances. Because the information contained in this book is of a general nature only, any reader who relies upon it does so at their own risk, and the author, publisher and contributors assume no responsibility under any circumstances. A medical practitioner should be consulted before beginning any new eating, exercise or health program.